A TRUE STORY OF MISDIAGNOSED/ UNEXPLAINABLE PAINS FOUND TO BE CAUSED BY TOBACCO USE

BY
Ferlin Clay Morgan

ISBN: 0-75961-590-X

This book is printed on acid free paper.

1stBooks – rev. 5/18/01

Acknowledgments go out to the following people:

Vascular Surgeon: Dr. William S. Dallas and Associates
Foot Doctor: Dr. Joe Southerland and Associates
Authors Wife: Jana L. Morgan
Authors Son: Nicholas C. Morgan
Authors Parents: Mr. & Mrs. James & Myrtle Morgan
Authors In-laws: Mr. & Mrs. George & Imogene Ivey

Well let me guess, your having a lot of body pains and a lot of other unexplainable things, that you have encountered too right. Such as:

1. Headaches
2. Leg Pain
3. Chest Pain
4. Back Pain
5. Foot Pain
6. Sinus Infection's
7. Nerve Trouble
8. Skin Rash
9. Can't sleep at night
10. No energy, feel drained all the time
11. Believe that you have Arthritis

The list goes on and on of course.

That's right you have taken enough medications to start your own drug store it seems like, and your still having all this pain, and your now thinking to yourself about all the doctor's you have seen for all these crazy pain's your having. By now your thinking, well just how many doctor's have I seen in the past. Let's see now! There's Dr. so and so-so and the doctor's that I can't even remember his or her name, and there's some doctor's that I don't even remember.

Well just set back and relax and take notes on this great story. I'm sure there will be something good in it for you and your family; maybe even your friends and neighbor's.

Let's Begin!

Ferlin Clay Morgan

I was a kid that was born in 1966 and was fairly healthy, and didn't have any sickness other than asthma trouble and as the year's past I seem to have grew out of it. I also didn't have any kind of birth defect's that I can recall of, when I was born. But in the late 1987 I began to encounter some complication's that I had never encountered before in my health, by that time I was about 21 year's of age. You got to remember that in those 21 years I run around, jumped and played just like any other kid. I played all kind's of sport's in school and out of school. I was named all conference in Basketball and Football, and I won the school's Physical Education Award for 8 years. Well I got out of school, I picked up all kinds of trades to get started in life with. Such things as a Mechanic, Carpenter work and operating heavy equipment, such as dozer's and loader's. I would go to work every day just like the next person, with no thoughts at all on my mind about getting down and not being able to work the next day. Now you have got to really think about this, I was only 21 years of age at the time this happened to me. I was quite along ways from home, and that really complicated things because I couldn't drive at the time and I didn't know where to begin to go and see a doctor, and I didn't know where I was going to find a hospital, and even if I could have there would still been a problem, because I didn't have the money to pay for a visit with a doctor.

I didn't have any insurance plan to pay the bills. I had one kind of insurance, and that was workman's comp. What I'm trying to say is that, I couldn't stand and tell a lie to my boss, doctor and friends, because it's like this, a few day's before I got down and couldn't walk, I was trying to make my way up on the dozer that I was operating and my

2

foot slipped off the edge of the track, and I hit my shin. I still worked that day, which I think that was on a Tuesday I worked Wednesday, but on a Thursday I had a little trouble, my shin or should I say the front lower part of my leg was swelled and was very sore and blue and I couldn't hardly walk, but I still worked that Thursday and Friday. Well a week or so past bye and I had recovered from my injury to my leg, and I thought everything was O.K., but guess what it wasn't over. About three week's later the really big trouble had arrived. This time it all began on a Wednesday morning, I was getting out of bed to go to work, and that's when I realized that I couldn't even dream of getting my sock or shoe on my left foot. My foot and ankle was so swelled, that I thought it was going to burst like bursting a balloon it sure looked bad, now as far as the pain goes, it wasn't that bad as long as I would keep my leg and foot elevated. But when I would drop it down to walk, that's when my foot felt like it was going to explode, but I had to stay calm and try to figure out why that my foot is swelled and what can I do about it.

Then it suddenly hit me, the only time swelling will occur without an injury, is when your circulation is really poor, that means that the flow of blood is trying to clot up in the deep artery vein, or a check valve in the Varicose Vein's is weak or is closing off due to inflammation in the Varicose Veins, then I began to wonder how could this happen, or why did this happen. Well anyway let's get back to where we were. All of this began on a Thursday morning and I knew if I could make it that day and all day Friday then I had my full work week in and I had it all whipped. What this means is that I would get a full weeks work without missing a day, and a chance of losing my job, and most of all I had to get somebody to drive me home to Tennessee, so I could get my family doctor to take a look at my swollen leg and foot. When this happened, I had friends and family in Georgia working to, and there were about three that were splitting rent with me, so you see I ask one of those old boys to drive me home in my car, and he said no problem, I can do that. The two days that I worked to finish my work week, I took Aspirin for a blood thinner and Extra Strength Tylenol for pain.

During my trip to come home to see my family, and to go see the doctor I had to ride in the back seat all the way, and the reason for that was if I had set in the front seat, I would have been setting up without a place to elevate my foot in the floor board, and that would cause me a lot of pain serious pain! I still had some pretty bad pain during my trip home due to all the swelling in my leg and foot, but regardless I still reached my home in Tennessee and I was certainly ready to get to my family doctor, and find out what could be causing all the swelling in my feet and legs, and the pain that it was causing me to have. My appointment to see my family doctor was, October 26, 1987. The doctor began treatment with cortisone injections in the leg tendon and gave me a prescription for Indomethacin. This pill was an anti-inflammatory medication, that was to help reduce swelling in my leg. The doctor also told me to keep warm moist heat on my leg about three to four times a day, and when I go to bed, try to keep my leg elevated up on pillows during the time that I am asleep, and to also do this during the time that I am not asleep.

According to the doctor my problem with my leg and foot swelling was as follows, blood clots in the superficial veins, and you know what that means, poor blood circulation in the leg and foot. The doctor had a name for this and it was Superficial Thrombophlbitis of the vein, goodness now that was a tongue twister wasn't it. Well anyways I had to return for a follow-up on the painful red streaks and very serious swelling that I had in my leg and foot and this visit was on November 14, 1987 and the doctor said that everything was looking a lot better, but I needed to continue with the Indomethacin for at least one more week, and to also continue the moist heat soakings on the leg and foot. My next visit to the doctor was on November 19, 1987 and the doctor decided to change my medication because the veins in my leg was trying to flare back up again. The medication that I had been taking was the Indomethacin, and the doctor changed it to Phenylbutazone, and I was to take this medicine for two weeks and that he would see me back in his office for a follow-up on this in about four to six weeks. Well, during that time, I had returned to work and I might have worked about two days and more bad luck had arrived, guess what, I was laid off from work and that was very bad timing because I had doctor bills and bank payments that had to be paid off. Check this out, as if bad luck hadn't caused me enough pain, the very two weeks that I had took off from work to get medical treatment on my leg, was the very two weeks I needed to be eligible for unemployment and that really got me upset, but that's part of life and I had to move on with my life, so I figured this would be a good time to get my leg back in top shape before I had to go back to the doctor in about a week. I continued to take medication and to elevate my leg up to increase blood circulation.

Well my next visit to the doctor was on December 7, 1987 and he told me that everything looks good and there isn't any swelling or redness in the lower leg and that he believes that the Phlabitis has resolved for now, and that he would give me one weeks prescription to take and if I had any trouble at all or if the Phlebitis returns, feel free to call his office for appointment. Well I took note to what the doctor told me, and I moved on with my life. About seven months had past, and as of phlebitis trouble goes, there was a few small lumps or blood clots in my leg at times and I would take and put moist heat pads on my leg for a little while and they would go away but, during the seven months that had past by, I encountered a new health problem, I broke out with a rash on my hand, arm, neck and forehead. I went to my doctor on July 16, 1988 and he told me that I had a fungus that is also called Tinea Corpus. The doctor gave me a prescription for a medication called Nizoral cream, that I was to apply this cream to the rash about three times a day for ten days or until its gone.

It took a little over two weeks, and the rash was gone but, according to the doctor during my follow-up on the rash, he said that this rash could return just as easy as before. Well I took the advise and left out to go back home. During the months of November 1988 through April 1989 I had to deal with sinus infections one after another plus the Phlebitis of the veins and the Tinea Corpus rash all together and it just about got the best of me, but I hung in there. I continued to deal with these problems through November 1989 until June 1991 the Phlebitis was pretty bad again and I had to go back to my doctor to get treatments again, and it would be just as before, the doctor gave me a few more Cortisone injections in the tender areas of the leg tendons I was also back in to see the doctor on July 1991 and August 1991 for the Phlebitis of the veins and just about all of the 1992 year I was in and out of the doctors office but, now there was one month of the 1992 year that I was in for something new. Very new to me, my lovely wife gave birth to our beautiful 6 pound 4 oz. Baby boy. I was so proud that I had know problem dealing with the pains and irritations that I was having at that time, but regardless of how I would like to have went on ignoring the pains and problems I was having, it was just impossible to do so. At the time my wife was in the hospital giving birth to our baby boy, I was dealing with another type of rash and it was very irritating I refused to go in and see the doctor, until I made sure my family was at home and they were comfortable, and then I went to see what the doctor thought this might have been. This rash was located on the upper lip, it was red, swollen and very sore.

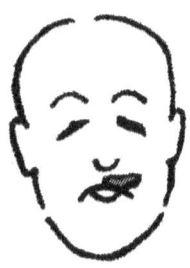

The doctor first tried some medicated lotion and some very good antibiotics for about ten days, and it just didn't seem to do the job, so when I went back to the doctor for a follow-up, he decided to change the medication, and go with something else, because the first medication just wasn't doing anything for the rash. So this time he had decided to try a cream called Bactraban and also a different kind of antibiotics for about ten more days and he told me if I had any trouble with this medication to get back to his office as soon as possible. I dealt with this rash from the last of August 1992 through the month of September and the month of October 1992, and it had finally healed up completely. I understood the doctor to say that this looked to be cellulites to him. That's just another name for an infection. The doctor also called this a simple skin fungus, and he said that I must be allergic to something that I was working in or around or that it could be something that I was eating or drinking or maybe it could be the pets that I'm around or even more he said it could even be my tobacco use also. By the time the doctor was finished, I guess you could say I was pretty confused. Well, I was very happy that it healed up, regardless of what the name of this skin rash might have been.

I was only interested in finding out what caused this and to try to do something about it. Let's see now I escaped the month of November 1992 without any rashes, but now I did have a little leg pain due to …the phlebitis of the vein in the leg, but my family and I still had a nice Thanksgiving Holiday. Now the month of December 1992 I encountered another type of pain. I was giving our little baby boy his bottle and it suddenly hit me, ouch! Guess what I had bent over to give the baby his bottle and my back popped and man did it hurt, it literally took my breath away. At this time I would like to say, if someone tells you that they are down in their back, don't just take them for granted, because it could be something very serious. They might have thrown a disc out in there back, and it easily could pinch a nerve down, and cause them to hurt really bad in their back and legs. That's all there is to it.

It's even possible to pinch a nerve in your back, and end up being paralyzed for a while or for life maybe. So do what my doctor told me to do, and that was not to be lifting and straining on objects that are much to heavy for me, according to my size and weight. He also told me to be careful, and not to over work my back what he meant by that was, if there was fifty rocks on one side of the yard and that needed to be moved to the other side of the yard don't try to move all fifty in one day. Break the work down into five days at ten rocks a day. Well, speaking for myself, I was that kind of person, I would try to move it all in one day. I, certainly took in consideration of what the doctor told me to do, because I had to lay down in bed and couldn't even get up without help, and let me tell you it still wasn't easy then. Anyways the doctor did give me some good advice and he gave me a prescription for Motrin I think, and Tylenol #3 with codeine for the pain. The doctor also had X-rays taken of my back and the results were very good, I hadn't ruptured any disc or broken anything, but the doctor said that I had a severely sprained back, and that I was also suffering with muscle spasms. That explains why that I couldn't get up and down hardly even if I had help. I had one follow-up on this and the doctor told me that I needed to wait a little longer before I started lifting and twisting or straining because he felt that even if I was feeling better that didn't mean that I was completely healed yet, I agreed with the doctor and he said to me, that if I needed to see him again to feel free to call his office for another appointment. In January 1993 I was in the doctor's office to get a shot, because I had stepped on a rusty nail, and it went about halfway through my foot and that wasn't good because I all ready had a history of phlebitis of the vein in the same leg.

That visit was the last time I had been to the doctor's office in nine months. I don't have any idea what had got into me, I guess it was that I was tired of taking medication and getting shots every time I turned around and most of all, was going to the lab to get blood work done, and then go back in about two days and let the lab tech do the blood work again for the second time in two days, "Why," well because the lab tech would call up and say, that the truck had broken down on the highway, when it was transporting the blood vials to a major testing lab, that runs these kind of test for the clinic that I was going to at that time. Looking back now, I must say that I was wrong for not going back to the doctor because I had a lot of trouble during that nine months that had past by. Let me tell you about some of these problems, such as, the sinus infections that I had was very painful. I've had sinus infections for a long, long time, and they continued to get worse. I would be pain free for a day or two and then all of a sudden my head would begin to hurt, then I would begin to get pressure in my face and then look out, I would encounter pain in my face and in my temples of my head and in my teeth my ears and in the back of my head that was excruciating pain.

"Anyways I thought so", because there was nothing that would stop it from hurting and it seemed like if I couldn't get it to stop the pain would get worse and worse by the seconds. I think every single person has a different experience with sinus trouble, and I respect that, but in the medical field, sinus is nothing but a simple thing called allergies, and there's a lot of people out there, men, women and children that suffer with allergies. Some of us were born with it right. Sometimes you will hear someone say that they were born with sinus trouble. Myself I believe that they are a lot of folks out there with sinus problems, and there's some out there with allergies and sinus trouble both. I believe truly myself that sinus is an allergie, and not all folks have allergies, because not everybody's sinuses is allergic to things such a trees and grass, pollen. But now for the ones who have the sinus allergy trouble, here's my theory and my advice on sinus allergies, I've had to deal with sinus allergies a good portion of my life and the type that I have are very, very painful. But I can't speak for everybody. There's the runny nose type of allergies, that a lot of people deals with every day. Here is what I think about the sinus allergies. I believe that sinus is an allergy and that when they flare up that the sinus cavity is trying to protect itself from getting infectious things such as tree, grass and pollen. We tend to say that we are allergic to certain things, but the sinus cavity is simply letting us know that it's not going to except these things. For a person that gets a runny nose and they think it's there sinuses, well that's true in a way. I believe that the sinus cavity will drain like this to flush themselves out, so that an infection can't set up and take over. What I am saying is, if the pollen got into the sinus cavity, and was left alone it would be considered as a germ, and that germ would fester up the sinus cavity, and then it could set up an infection. But if

11

your immune system is strong enough, it could easily begin to take over and suddenly it would produce rapid amounts of mucus through the sinus cavity to flush the sinus cavity out. I also believe that the sinus is nothing but a little filter that catches the dust and anything else that we breath such as the tree and grass pollen, but now if your immune system is weak, then it's not going to produce the mucus that flushes out the sinus cavity. Let's see if I can explain something without getting everyone confused. Here we go, there are two kinds of sinus allergies, there is the kind that when they begin to act up they tend to drain a lot with a rapid amount of mucus, now I also think that some people are allergic to the things I talked about earlier, and that was such things as grass and tree pollen, I think that the mucus continues to drain until whatever is irritating the sinus cavity is washed out by the mucus that our good old immune system produces. These kind of allergy victims, need to be aware of things that cause them to have trouble with there sinus allergies, here is a few things to remember, in the spring time when the pollen levels are very high, try to wear a filtered mask when your out doors working, and also avoid such things as pollen, mold, dust, hay and extreme dry heat, or anything that you remember that bothered you before. Now the other type of sinus allergies is the kind that a lot of folks have real bad pain with. People that have these kind of sinus allergies will do anything to get there head to stop hurting them. The sinus allergies that these people have, began just like the others did. They had a runny nose a lot, or at least until the allergies went away. I know this because this is how my sinus allergies began. The pain that I was having with my sinus allergies was a sinus infection. I also think this happen to me because my immune system was down. The reason why? Was, because I was sick and I wasn't eating like I should have. Now when your immune system is down you are at a very high risk of getting many kinds of sickness. I was a smoker and that is a bad thing for sinus allergy victims, because it continues to irritate the sinus cavity. Even if your immune system is working, it would be fighting a losing battle, the sinus is a little filter to catch the dust and everything else that we breath, and if it is full of smoke all the time, the nose is it going to do what it was created to do. It can't because it's full of smoke, let me tell you something else, when you continue to have the smoke in the sinus cavity the nicotine causes infection to set up. It's as simple as this, the immune system can only produce so much mucus to wash out the little sinus cavity, filter, and if we continue to fill it with smoke, then how do we plan on healing the sinus cavity. Let me tell you something that I have learned first hand, when you get a sinus infection, it is very hard to get rid of it, and even when you do it takes a good bit of time to heal the sinus cavity. It took me about 2 ½ to 3 months after I quit smoking to heal my sinus cavities and I am glad its all over, because I don't have the sinus infections anymore, and I don't have to suffer with the bad pain that comes with it either. My sinuses don't bother me anymore, by drying out and giving me all the bad pain that I was having in my head. You must remember, I didn't say that my sinuses, healed up and got better over night or in a week or so. It just don't work out that easy. First of all if you are a smoker you must begin by, quitting the cigarette smoking, simply because the smoke will continue to keep the sinuses infected and very tender. Step two, is if you are dealing with an infection at this time, try to get yourself an appointment with your doctor to see if it's possible to get something for the pain. That is if you are having pain with the sinus infection, and you will also need a prescription for some type of antihistamine to relieve the symptoms of the sinus allergy, this works by blocking the effects of histamine. Also, the doctor may give you a nasal spray called, vancenase this is used to open up the infected sinus cavity, because it tends to dry up and tighten up and it causes you to have severe pain. The nasal spray is used to put moister back in the sinus cavity so that it will begin to drain and ease the pain. Step three, is to continue use of the nasal moisturizing spray, but not the prescription sprays such as vecenace, beconace and vancenace, because these types of nasal sprays are believed to be addictive. I use a nasal spray that can be found at your local pharmacy, drug store or you can do like me. I just go to Wal-mart's and purchase about three bottles at a time, of the Saline Nasal Spray.

This is a nasal moisturizing spray. It can be purchased in a 1.5 fl. Oz. Bottle only. It contains sodium chloride 0.65% phenylocorbinol as a preservative. It also contains purified water, and sodium bicorbonate. Here is one little reminder, to you before I leave the subject of sinus allergies. Remember to use the Saline Nasal Spray, once in the morning once in the evening and once before bed time, continue this sequence for the first month, and then reduce the sequence to once in the morning and once in the evening. Spray twice in each nostril during every dosage. You should also remember to keep this and all drugs out of the reach of children.

I also, had to deal with the flu bug, sore throat, toothache, earache, and that good old spring time sinus trouble. Also, along about July 1993 I began to have trouble with the phlebitis in my right leg. Did you catch on to what I said about the phlebitis in my right leg. Well if you haven't, then just think for a moment, the first time the phlebitis flared up it was in the left leg, and this time, it just so happens to be in the right leg. And what this tells me is that the phlebitis is moving around, and that isn't good. Phlebitis is nothing but a simple blood clot, and this could very well turn loose and go to my lungs and possible choke me to death while I'm asleep. These clots that I was having, were located in the Varicose vein, these are the little veins that we can see in our arms and legs. These clots will usually form where there's restriction in the artery wall, because the blood can't flow smoothly, when you have a restriction in the artery or vein the blood flow slows down, and most of the time it will clot up against a little muscle called a check valve, that is also found in the Varicose artery or vein. Now it has been said that if one of these blood clots makes it up to the groin area, it could easily dump over into the deep artery, called the deep femoral and this could spell trouble, because the blood clot could easily go straight to your heart and kill you. I always believed that my smoking habit, was the cause of me having what the doctor called phlebitis, but now listen here I was just like the next man or women, I would defend my smoking habit because I simply couldn't quit smoking.

I always said, that if I could get some good concrete evidence, that my smoking was causing my trouble, I would find a way to quit smoking. But up to this point, I had not found any concrete proof of this yet. But now let me tell ya something, I couldn't give up hope, I just continued on searching for answers to all my health problems, and also learn how to deal with the new ones, such as the time in August 1993 when I had the real bad chest pains, I mean to say that these pains that I was having in my chest were really bad. It would literally make me drop to my knees. This would hurt me in my chest, and both of my arms. It also made me light headed and jerky all over, inside and out. And I would get real bad sick at my stomach, and this seem to be getting worse all the time. I took my chest pains to the doctor as fast as possible.

After the doctor finished giving me an examination, he said that he just flat out could not find anything that could be causing my problems, other than the Chronic peptic disease, that I had. He gave me some sample packs of Tagament 400mg that I was to take for two weeks. He ask that I call, in two weeks when I finished the medication, and if the Tagamet has helped, then he will issue a prescription for maintenance therapy with Tagamet. The doctor also had some blood work taken on me and I had to run by the near by hospital to get several x-rays taken. I had to wait a few days on the X-rays and the blood work, but regardless, the reports finally returned to my doctor, and he told me that the results were negative. That means that they, nor my doctor couldn't find anything that would be causing the chest pain, dizziness and feeling jerky all over. The x-rays and blood work showed nothing of any type of ulcers or hernia and there was very mild findings of peptic disease within the stomach. So I guess that I will just do what I was told, and that was, if I needed to see the doctor for anything, please feel free to call and set up an appointment, and that was just what I did, but this time it's something that we are familiar with and that is the phlebitis of the vein. Let's see now the last time that the phlebitis flared up on me was in July 1993 and here it is December 1993 and its back, I must admit it isn't no where near as bad as what it was the last time I was bothered by it. The doctor gave me a prescription for Indomethacin 25mg to take for two weeks, and yes the swelling most definitely went down, but as strangely as it may sound, I had some red knots to flare up on the inner side of my ankles, and let me say this, if you have ever mashed a finger or toe, then you can say that you have experienced what it feels like if you have never dealt with phlebitis of the vein. This last little encounter of phlebitis that I had, returned on March 1994 and that was only three months later since that last experience with the phlebitis had occurred. So much for talking about the last time I had a visit with the doctor over the phlebitis problem that I had. I think it was March 3, 1994 that I was just in for a visit with the doctor, because of some small painful phlebitis knots on the inner sides of my ankles, and now here I am back in the doctors office again. Only this time it was more than just the phlebitis. It was several things this time. As the doctor was giving me an examination this is what he said to me. Your history is rather vague and wondering. You say for the past seven years or so you have been having pain and swelling in the lower legs and ankles, but over the past three months it has gotten worse. You have been complaining of pain and swelling in both ankles, and that you barely can walk when you arise out of bed in the mornings.

You also are saying that the only thing that seems to help is, hot water soaks. The doctor also was aware of the superficial phlebitis in the lower legs, and for a long time I had to wear men's support hoses on regular basis for this. Over the past three or four months I had developed pain in the extreme lower part of my back and posterior hip. My knees had been swelling up on me at times, and I was also having pain in my shoulders, hands and wrist. I had no weight loss, no fevers that I can think of. I also had broken out with a chronic rash on my arms, neck and the top of my foot. During my visit with the doctor, he had some blood work obtained to include a chemistry panel, CBC, westergren sed rate, ANA, rheumatoid factor, and C-reactive protein. I was given lcc of cortistat- 10 and lcc of Cortistat Laim. I was also treated for Tenia with a combination of Nizoral 200mg tablets and take 1 tablet a day for 10 days. Plus I was treated with the Nizoral cream at the same time. Also for ten days, twice a day. I was given an outpatient request for X-rays of the LS spine, sacroiliac joints and both ankles. The exam that was requested to check for arthritis is LS spine and both ankles S.L.J. had returned and here is the results. Normal radiographic examination of the left ankle an AP, lateral and oblique views. There was also a small discussion about a rounded benign appearing 1 cm lucency within the anterior aspect of the calcareous. There was no arthritic changes delineated on either ankle in response to a clinical question in that regard. Normal radiographic examination of the lumbar-sacral spine in frontal, lateral and cones down views of the lumbar-sacral joints. Both S I joints appeared to be widely patent with no abnormal areas of indistinctness or increased sclerosis evident. No cystic areas are noted. The doctor also told me that the impression that he gets is, that there is no abnormality identified. Hard to believe isn't it. After getting all kinds of X-rays taken and blood work sent off to a special lab to be tested for just about every possible thing, that could be thought of. And still I had not gotten a single answer for all the different body pains that I was having, and this was bad news for me, because this pain wasn't a past time pain. It simply was a continuous pain that would never let up. I wanted to make sure that these blood test results could be seen by every one, and to also let you know that all the X-rays had returned and they were all said to be normal. I believe that folk's will be very surprised when they find out what was causing all of my trouble.

Especially after finding out that the X-rays that were taken, was all normal and after seeing and reading the blood test results for themselves, and to find that they were all normal to. Here are the blood test results that I talked about. Blood work was collected on or about March 9, 1994 and the results had returned to my doctor on or about March 11, 1994. Here are the results: TEST REQUEST: cbc, sed rate-wetergren, c-reative protein, ra latex agglutinat., ana (Hep-2), acp, hdl.

ADDITIONAL INFORMATION:

Test Name	Normal Results	Abnormal Results	Unit	Reference Range
Lipids:				
Cholesterol	158		MG/DL	130-200
Triglycerides	50		MG/DL	30-200
HDL	36		MG/DL	30-75
Chol/HDL	4.4			
LDL Chol (Calculated)	112		MG/DL	0-130
Desirable: Less than 130 Mg/Dl				
Borderline-High:131-159 Mg/Dl				
High:greater than 160 Mg/Dl				
Protein:				
Protein-total-Serum	7.1		GM/DL	6.0-8.5
Albumin	4.5		G/DL	3.5-5.5
Globulin	2.6		G/DL	2.0-3.5
A/G Ratio	1.7			1.0-2.4
CBC:				
WBC	8.0		X10-3D/ML	3.7-10.5
RBC	5.05		X10-6/ML	4.1-5.6
HGB	15.1		GM/DL	12.5-17.0
HCT:	44.3		%	36-50
MCV	88		Femtoliters	80-98
MCH	29.9		Picograms	27-34
MCHC	34.1		%	33-35
NEUT	69		%	40-74
LYMPH	22		%	14-46

A True Story of Misdiagnosed/Unexplainable Pains
Found to be Caused by Tobacco Use

Test Name	Normal Results	Abnormal Results	Unit	Reference Range
CBC:				
Monocytes	5		%	4-13
EOS	3		%	0-3
Platelet Count	184		X10-3/MM-3	155-385
Sed Rate-Westergren:				
Sed Rate-Westergren	2		MM/HR	0-20
SED RATE NORMAL RANGES:				
MALE (UNDER 50) 0-15 MM/HR				
MALE (OVER 50) 0-20 MM/HR				
C-Reactive Protein:				
C-Reactive Protein:	NEG		Negative	
RA Latex AGG	NEG		Negative	
ANA (Hep-2):				
ANA	NEG		Negative	
REFERENCE VALUES FOR ANA:				
NORMAL: NEGATIVE AT LESS THAN 1:40				
DILUTION BY IFA ASSAY.				
ANA Titer	Not Indicated			
ACP, HDL:				
Glucose	104		MG/DL	65-115
BUN	12		MG/DL	7-25
Creatinine	0.9		MG/DL	0.6-1.5
Sodium – Serum	143		MEQ/L	135-147
Potassium	4.2		MEQ/L	3.5-5.3
Choloride (Serum)	104		MEQ/L	96-109

Test Name	Normal Results	Abnormal Results	Unit	Reference Range
ACP, HDL:				
Uric Acid – Serum	4.1		MG/DL	3.9-9.0
Calcium (Tot-Serum)	9.6		MG/DL	8.5-10.8
Phosphorus-Serum	3.0		MG/DL	2.5-4.5
ALK.PHOS	66		U/L	25-140
SGOT	18		U/L	0-40
SGPT	19		U/L	0-45
LDH (Serum)	122		U/L	0-240
Bilirubin (Total)	0.4		MG/DL	0.1-1.2
GGT	18		U/L	0-65
Iron	62		MCG/DL	40-200

As you can see, all of the test results were negative. Come on and hang in there because this story is just getting started, you think it's interesting now, well you just keep reading and you will really find it to be interesting. It was around March 25, 1994 when my doctor's decided to try something different, and that was to send me to see an Orthopedic surgeon, and that they did. My doctor's set me up with an Orthopedic surgeon about 56 miles from my home, and I went over to my appointment and guess what, they turned me away because they didn't except my insurance, and when they told me that they wouldn't take me in because of my insurance, that really bothered me because I was 56 miles from home and I was in some very serious pain. So I thought I would ask them if they would except cash, you are not going to believe this.

They said no to cash. You know why, because they told me that they were under a contract with the state to participate in the state insurance plan. And that was the kind of insurance that I had, and as far as I am concerned that is one bad mark against the state insurance so, remember this part of this story because it comes into play later in this story. But anyway I did return home to give the news to my doctors and to see what was next for me. My doctor said to me that they would like to apologize for all the trouble and for the trip that I made for nothing, and that they would like to try and get me an appointment with another Orthopedic surgeon, and about all that I would or could say was, whatever. I was in a lot of pain, and I didn't really care either way, but they did just what they said they would do, and that was to get me in to see some other Orthopedic doctor. So my doctor's found an Orthopedic doctor that would take my insurance, and right away the appointment was set up for me, and that was the following day of when I was turned away because of the kind of insurance I had. This new appointment was set up on or around May 2, 1994 and when it was time to go, I picked up some new X-rays that had been taken of my back, hips, and feet. I headed out to retrieve a brand new opinion of what is causing all of my body pains. This is what the orthopedic surgeon said about me, during the examination that he gave me on May 2, 1994, I was a 28 year old patient that was seen by my family doctors on or around March 9, 1994 at which they made a diagnosis of synovitis in my ankles and, I also had a fungus infection on several areas of the body, such as the forearms, hands and feet, and I also had a history of superficial phlebitis in the left lower leg. I was given some Cortisone injections in which I stated was very painful. I was also given some Nizoral for my fungus infection and was referred for X-rays, also my doctors sent a copy of my records and laboratory tests and all of the X-ray reports on me, to the Orthopedic surgeon. The X-rays of both ankles and the lumbar spine including the sacroiliac joints, were reported to be normal, my laboratory tests for arthritis, including a sedimentation rate, C-reactive protein, RA test, ANA test, were all normal. My blood count was normal. Uric acid was normal. Over just a few days time I had complained to my doctor about hurting in my neck, my shoulders, my wrist, my hands, my hips, my knees, and my ankles. I also had a lot of stomach burn with some nausea and vomiting, I also would spit up blood sometimes. I would have migraine headaches with neck pain that was deadly, I would have chest pains at times due to some type of arthritis in my chest bone. I had no history of any serious injuries or operations. The Orthopedic Examined me, and he said that there was tenderness about my knees, but no effusion.

He also said that there was tenderness about both ankles. There was swelling mainly on the medial aspect of the left ankle and foot around the posterior tibial tendon. He also found diffuse tenderness in the posterior cervical, dorsal, and the lumbar spine, and down over the sacrum. There was no reflex changes or atrophy in the lower extremities. The Orthopedic surgeon also found that my back motions were limited to about 20% and somewhat painful. He said that my chest expansion was 3 inches. After the Orthopedic doctor had finished a full examination on me he left the room for a short few minutes., and then he returned, the doctor handed me some literature to read, and he also took time to tell me what he believed was causing, me all the different kinds of pain. He said he felt that I had a form of tenosynovitis, also known to be inflammation of the tendon sheath.

Tenosynovitis is the name given when the tendons become bound in an inflammatory mass. The doctor also said that I had what he believed to be, was fibromyalgia arthritis related disease. Your most likely thinking the same thing that I was, about what in this world is fibromyalgia arthritis. I will tell you more about this kind of arthritis, after the orthopedic surgeon finishes with his diagnosis and treatment that he performed on me. He has already given his diagnosis of me and now here is the treatments that he performed on me. The doctor gave me several injections in the lumbosacral area, that is the extreme lower part of my back, and the tendon sheath of the posterior tibial tendon also known as the arched area of the foot. The medication that was used in the injections, was 10mg of Kenalog and some Xylocaine. The doctor also gave me an elastic support to wear on my left ankle. I was already wearing a pair of men's support hoses, because of my previous superficial thrombophlebitis.

The kind of medicine treatment that the Orthopedic surgeon felt that I needed to be taking, was not just one but several. The doctor said that he would let my own family doctors have a copy of his medical records on me, and a list of the medication that he felt that I needed to be taking. I had an appointment set up for May 31, 1994 and I had to have it changed to June 6, 1994 to see my family doctors. This visit is a follow-up on what the Orthopedic doctor had to say about me. When I finally made it to my doctors office, he reminded me about what the Orthopedic surgeon said that he felt was my problem, and what kind of medication that I should be treated with. Well to begin with my doctor reviewed my records he received from the Orthopedic surgeon and then he began to tell me about what the results were. My doctor said that he is aware of the trigger point injections in the low back and the arched area of the feet. He also told me that the Orthopedic doctor diagnosed me, to have an arthritis related disease, called fibromyalgia and also a disease called tenosynovitis. He also spoke to me about the trigger point injections and wanted to know if I was feeling any better at all. I told him that it helped ease the pain for about 24 to 48 hours and then it returned just as painful as it was, before the injections took place. My doctor was also aware of the educational material that the Orthopedic surgeon gave me to read up on, so that I could get a better understanding of the fibromyalgia disease. My doctor found that I had a lot more than just a basic understanding of the fibromyalgia disease. The Orthopedic surgeon also gave me a prescription for Ativan – 1mg to help me sleep better, and it didn't help me very much at all to be truthful about it. And that's just what I told my family doctor. Before I tell you what kind of medications that my doctor used to begin treatments for this disease. I'm going to take a little time to tell more about the disease called fibromyolgia arthritis. The facts, Fibromyalgia originally named fibrositis meaning connective tissue inflammation the syndrome is a common form of chronic generalized muscular pain and fatigue. In recent years its name had been changed to reflect the finding that it does not involve inflammation of the tissues, but rather unexplained pain (myalgia) in them. Still the names are often used interchangeably.

People with fibromyalgia may experience deep muscular aching, throbbing, burning or stabbing and a feeling of being completely drained of energy. Pain is often worst at "tender points" in specific locations on the body, although some people may not be aware of that until they are examined by a doctor. Other common symptoms include disturbances in deep-level sleep, headaches, chest pain, menstrual cramps, dizziness and irritable lowel syndrome, which is characterized by alternate constipation and diarrhea, bloating and abdominal pain.

However painful and fatiguing, fibromyalgia does not appear to cause permanent damage to the connective tissue or organs, and it doesn't lead to deformation like many other forms of arthritis. Symptoms often wax and wane, and may become worse during times of illness or stress or often excessive physical exertion. Unlike inflammatory forms of arthritis, which can be confirmed by X-rays, fibromyalgia produces no obvious signs. X-rays are normal. Routine blood tests to detect or measure such factors as white and red cell count, sedimentation rate, antinuclear antibodies and rheumatoid factor – are all negative in most of these people. People with fibromyalgia have a lot of symptoms for which doctors can't find an obvious cause, "and often when doctors can't find and organic cause, they tend to think there must be apsychological one. Although there is not yet a cure or even a clear understanding of the condition or its cause – experts say some recent developments are definitely a step in the right direction. By now your thinking to your, wondering if this could be your aches and pain problem.

It's very much possible. But now listen here, there's a small catch, to having the disease called fibromyalgia arthritis. To meet the diagnostic criteria for fibromyalgia, a person must have widespread pain in all four quadrants of the body that has lasted for at least three months and tenderness in at least 11 of the 18 specified tender points of the body. Although there is no laboratory test to confirm a fibromyalgia diagnosis, negative test results can sometimes rule out other causes of pain and fatigue, and thus lead a doctor that's familiar with fibromyalgia, to suspect the syndrome. Because many of the symptoms of fibromyalgia may be similar to those of other illnesses, including rheumatoid arthritis and lupus, gout, jet leg and others, it's important to seek treatment from a doctor knowledgeable in arthritis-related diseases. If you don't already have such doctor, then your local Chapter of Arthritis Foundation can provide a referral. I think the hottest theory of research looks at the central nervous system, and particularly how neural hormones affect pain and fatigue. Neural are said to be the chemical messengers of the central nervous system that plays a role in such functions as sleep, pain sensation, immunity, the constriction and dilation of blood vessels, and even your emotions believe it or not. Because fibromyalgias cause is not known, current treatments are geared to easing the painful symptoms of the disease rather than curing it. Among the most common is the use of drugs called tricyclic antidepressants to promote deeper sleep. That seems to be important to try to help the sleep disturbance, although improving sleep doesn't completely alleviate fibromyalgia symptoms. Other treatments include use of nonsteroidal ani-inflammatory drugs and analgesics to improve muscle pain, relaxation techniques to help reduce muscle tension, and injection of local anesthetic into the tender points. Also here are some of the medication treatments that the Orthopedic surgeon told my doctor that he felt that I needed to be taking for the treatment of the fibromyalgia arthritis. As follows, beginning with paxil 20mg tablet, dispense 30, one q.a.m., Amitriptylline 25mg q.d. dose after supper, first week one tab., second week two tabs, third week three tabs, fourth week four tabs. Both of these medication were used to help me sleep more at night, because I wasn't resting very well when I would go to sleep these two medication were supposed to relax the nervous system. The paxil itself, wasn't doing nothing for me. But when I had to begin taking the Amitriptyline, then I was in for a whole new experience. Let me tell you this, they made me so sleepy that I couldn't hold up, and when I got my sleep out or over with, I think it would be safe to say that I had the worst hang over head ache that anyone could possible encounter. That didn't last to long with me if you know what I mean. I had to flat out quit them simply because they was doing me as much harm as they was good. Next on the list of medications was, Extra Strength Tylenol caplets 500mg t.i.d. for pain. This wasn't any good for me either, because it's like this, if the pain that I was having, was measured on a pain scale from 1to 10, it would definitely be a 10 with no questions ask, and with the pain that I was having, I believe that if I had taken the whole complete bottle at the time of troubles I just don't think it would made a difference, but anyways this wasn't the last of the medication, there was also a medication that I had to take for a hernia that was irritating my stomach, and that was the Tagamet form stomach pill, they were 400mg, dispense, one daily after supper. I did this for one month.

My doctor said he wasn't for sure this would work but I guess we can try and see. The Orthopedic doctor seem to think that I would notice some improvement over a period of three months on this treatment plan. But he also told my family doctor that he couldn't guarantee just how much improvement. My doctor also said to me that this is a chronic problem; however it tends not to be a crippling type of disorder. I was to return to my family doctors office on monthly visits. My family doctor told me if there was no improvement in three months that he would send me back to see the Orthopedic surgeon. I did return for the first follow-up on the three month medication therapy that my family doctor had me on. This follow-up was July 8, 1994, and the results was simple. There was no change in the cramps and pain that I was having. My second follow-up was August 9, 1994 one month later, and guess what, very little change.

At this time my weight had dropped from 142 to 135, but the pain had eased a little, and my appetite was a little better, even though I had lost five pounds over the past month. I was still complaining of profound morning stiffness and burning pain in my legs which resolves after a period of activity and after taking the Ibuprofen. But still no change in energy level. The activity that I was talking about was massaging of the leg and arm muscles and very little walking. If I did to much walking in which I couldn't do, it would cause my legs to lock up or cramp up and I couldn't walk. The pain that I would get in my legs was extremely bad. On a pain scale from 1 to 10, I would say that it was a 10 with no doubt in my mind. I did try some exercising but it made my pain worse and I had to quit. I tried riding a bicycle and that didn't seem to help. I was taking hot water soaks twice a day and this would help for a little while, and then the pain would return. At this time I could not eat much at all, my appetite was very poor, my weight would go up and down a lot. My weight would be 130 pounds this week and the following week it would be 140 pounds, then I could give it, another week and my weight would drop down to 128 pounds. My blood pressure would usually stay around 100/70. I felt bad all the time, didn't have much energy for nothing, I stayed sleepy all the time, but as strange as it may sound, I could try to sleep and couldn't. I brought this up to my doctor during my next appointment with him. The doctor seem to think that the problem that I was having with my sleep pattern, was the fibromyalgia arthritis. The doctor told me, that he wants me to try a new medication, the name of this was paxil. The doctor said this should help me sleep a little better. He also told me to start, taking a mid-day nap if I could, and to see if it made me feel any better. It did just that, but it only helped a little. I still felt bad all the time, and stayed sleepy a lot. But I did what the doctor told me to do. The doctor also ask me to stay clear of all caffeine products. He gave me a prescription for paxil 20mg / Amitriptyline 50mg./ Ibuprofen 800mg./ Tagament 800mg. Diphenhydramine 25mg. This last visit with my doctor was around October 6, 1994. He also said that he believes that I need to be seen by a rheumatoligist consultant. I returned to my family doctor for a follow-up on or about November 9, 1994 for my diffuse pains that I was having I had a history of bad pains for most of the past twelve years, in my legs and arms. This pain began to increase and spread to different areas as time past by.

31

That includes areas such as my ankles, calves, legs, hips, low back, upper back, shoulders and arms, and these pains prevented me from doing most of anything. At times I would be in so much pain, that it would bring tears to my eyes. It would bother me like this even if I had taken my medications. I had seen an orthopedist in the past for all the pains I had been having, it was he who injected a couple of areas, with cortisone which were better temporarily and then got worse in a couple of days. I had decided that there was no cure out there for me, because I felt that my family doctor had tried just about everything possible, between the medication and all the doctors that I had seen in the past, I was convinced that there wasn't any cure for me, you see. It just seemed like a bad dream, but trust me it wasn't. It just got worse. I got to the point to where it seemed like I was in to see my doctor or doctors about every day. I also was getting to the point to where I couldn't hardly walk, because of the pains and cramps I was having. These pains just seem to get worse from day to day. To be honest about it, I got to wondering if I would ever find a doctor out there in this world that could tell me what was causing my pains and cramps. I began to venture out to see other doctors, after hearing my doctor say that he just didn't know what I had and that he was going to be retiring soon and that I would need to begin seeing another doctor in his clinic or a doctor elsewhere. So that left me between a rock and a hard place. At that time I was on the state insurance plan and everyone was assigned to a doctor or clinic of your choice, for one year, and you just couldn't run out and see any doctor you are not assigned to unless your doctor agreed to refer you to another doctor. So I continued to do so for a few more months. Since

November 1994 I had been in to see the doctor numerous of times. Let's see! I saw the doctor of my choice January 1995 and this continued right on through February, March, April, May, June and July of 1995 and let me tell you I was in some bad, I'm talking bad pain.

This stuff would bring tears in my eyes, and let me say this much. I just don't shed tears for nothing. I once had a farm tractor to set down on my thumb and I patiently set the jack back under it and raised it up off of my thumb. Yes it hurt like crazy but I didn't shed a tear. Now does that tell you anything about what I was dealing with from day to day. I was having all this bad pain, and was still getting up every morning and going out to work. I did this to get my mind off things like the pain I was having and to relieve all the stress I was having, this would also give my wife and little boy a break too, because I would be kind of cranky around them and not meaning to be. But they learned to try, and ignore me, even though it was hard, for them to do so. But they also knew that it was their support, that kept me encouraged not to quit trying to find the answers to all the sickness and pains that I was having. I really didn't have much of a choice. I had to keep trying, to find answers, because the pain was so bad, that it had me literally suicidal. The pains and red streaks that I was having would break loose and move around but trust me, there was never any signs of healing or any pain relief for me. I believe it was around July 3, 1995, that I had to get my wife to call and get me an appointment with the doctor. The reason why, was that I had encountered something new, about what I had going on with my legs. When I got in to see the doctor, I told him about the new flare ups that were located on the inner sides of the right thigh just above the knee. I was also complaining of dependent redness of the foot and pain and swelling about the area of the right great toe. I had some swelling and tenderness in the area of the first MPP joint of the right great toe. I had no calf tenderness. This went on for another week, with no change. My doctor's said that they were going to rule out gout, as one of the possibilities, that they thought was causing all these flare ups of blood clots in my legs. The doctors requested a serum uric acid test. They also set me up for daily whirlpool visits for about five days. The doctor had me to continue to wear the support hose for men. He also told me to stay off the leg, and keep it elevated. The doctor gave me a prescription of Indomethicin 25mg one a day, plus Tylenol #3 dispense 30, one or two at a time for leg pain. As strange as it may sound, my doctors continued to treat me for my troubles and pain, but it just seem to never do any good. My family doctors decided that I needed to go to a vascular surgeon, during my last visit in August of 1995. They also told me that there wasn't much more they could offer me, from a medical standpoint. I was also told that I could not continue to take Indomethocin on a regular basis because of the possibility of bone marrow depression.

This was something that I was already familiar with, but that is quite alright, because we can never get enough of good advice right. Well anyway, the doctors told me that I also needed to continue to wear the men support hose on my legs, and they would try to get me an appointment set up with vascular surgeon. Here we go again, test more test and X-rays to send to the vascular surgeons office. About September of 1995 was when the most recent test were taken. Guess what? About two and a half to three days past and the doctors office called to see if I would come back in and let them do all the blood work again. They said that the truck had broken down and all the specimens had thawed out and, that they couldn't be used for testing. So I went back to the lab. Just as I was ask to. Let me say this! It doesn't feel good to be poked to death with needles, but it is something that's got to be done for our own sake sometimes. All of my test that were sent off to the lab, came back to say normal results, as you can see on this chart.

TEST REQUEST: CBC WITH DIFFERENTIAL & PLATELET, PROTHROMBIN (QUANTITATIVE), PLASMA, ACTIVATED PARTIAL THROMBOPLASTIN TIME (APTT), ANTI-THROMBIN III, PLASMA, PROTEIN C AND PROTEIN S ANTIGENS, PLASMA,

ADDITIONAL INFORMATION:
PATIENT TYPE: COLLECT TIME (MIN): 00

Test Name	Normal Results	Abnormal Results	Unit	Reference Range
CBC WITH DIFFERENTIAL & PLATELET:				
WBC	7.0		Thous/MM3	3.7-10.5
RBC	4.71		Mill/MM3	41.-5.6
Hemoglobin	14.5		G/DL	12.5-17.0
Hematocrit	42.1		%	36.0-50.0
MCV	89		FL	80-98
MCH	30.8		PG	27-34
MCHC	34.4		%	32-36
RDW	13.1		%	11.7-15.0
Neutrophils	64		%	40-74
Lymphocytes	28		%	14-46
Monocytes	5		%	4-13
Eosinophils	3		%	0-7
Basophils	0		%	0-3
Platelet Count	209		Thous/MM3	155-385
PROTHROMBIN TIME:				
INR	1.20 Low			2.0-3.0
Patient PT	12.9		Seconds	10.0-25.0
Normal Patient Mean	12.0		Seconds	
Ratio	1.1			

NOTE: THE PT RATIO IS DERIVED BY DIVIDING THE PATIENT'S P.T. BY THE NORMAL (NON-MEDICATED) POPULATION MEAN.

Normal Range:	PT	10.5-14.0
Therapeutic Ranges	PT	20.0-25.0
	INR	2.0-3.0
	INR *	2.5-3.5

*(PresenceOf Mechanical PROSTHETIC VALVES OR RECURRENT SYSTEMIC EMBOLISM))

Copies of all test were sent to the Vascular surgeons office. The reason for this was that I was to be seen by the Vascular doctor for a illness called Superficial Phlebitis.

Here is what the Vascular doctor had to say about me. This 29 year old gentlemen gives a history of left leg superficial phlebitis as far back as 1988. He developed some superficial phlebitis in his right medial calf last fall. This has improved with cortisone injections. He does not have much in the way of swelling. It is tender along the medial aspect of his calf. He has never had a DVT that he is aware of. He is a smoker, and I was a bad smoker. The doctor also stated that he had received the lab reports that my family doctor had performed including a normal sed rate, A&A, CBC. Lipids and protein were also within normal limits he said. Creative protein was negative. I was on Ibuprofen at this time. During the time that the Vascular surgeon gave me an examination, I must admit that, I was nervous of what he might find out or what he may need to do to get this under control. For an example, the surgeon may want to strip the superficial veins from my legs. But I stayed calm until the doctor did the examination and gave me his opinion of what he thought my problem was with my legs. This is the Vascular Surgeon's opinion after he did the examination. The doctor said that I had no edema of either the right or left lower extremities. He said that I had a few scattered Varicosities in the left calf but other wise unremarkable. He said that I had fairly good circulation of the right foot with palpable posterior tibial and dorsalis pedis pulses. That's pulses in the feet and toes. There was a cord which feels Chronic palpable or you could say a small blockage, in the mid and upper medial calf, probably along the course of the greater Saphenous vein consistent with superficial phlebitis. There were no evidence of infection. It was mildly tender. No popliteal masses are noted. There was no edema or calf tenderness otherwise. The Vascular doctors impression or opinion of what he thought was my problem with my legs, was the same old thing that I had heard before, and that was superficial thrombo-phlebitis. This is known to be recurrent. That means that you can treat it, and if it clears up, for some odd reason it would always return again. The doctors recommendation was that I didn't have involvement with deep venous system and he said that he would like to obtain a noninvasive lower extremity study. In addition, the doctor said that he thinks that it would be wise for me to discontinue my smoking habit, as this may have some contributing factor. During this time of my life, it would have been hard to stop smoking, reason why was that I was very stressed out and I was in a lot of pain, and I also felt like that I was going to die just about anytime, but I didn't. If I had known then what I know now, the smoking habit would have been history. Well back to what the doctor was saying, and that was that he also thought it is also reasonable to obtain a CBC, PT/PTT, protein C and S, anti-thrombin 3 and fibrinagen levels to be sure that I did not have some type of couagulopathy. He also thought that I should discontinue the Ibuprofen as I have been on it a long time and should begin taking one aspirin per day. The doctor said that he wants me to walk on a regular basis. Copies of these results were forwarded to my family doctors office. The vascular surgeon told me that he would see me any time or on referral. This visit took place on or about July 24, 1995. A few days past and the vascular surgeons office called and said that they had set me up for a doctors appointment to have a lower Extremity Venaus Evaluation by Doppler radar. This works just like the machine that is used to monitor a women's pregnancy.

This machine is called an ultrasound machine. I was evaluated with a history of superficial phlebitis of the vein, in the right leg. This has been present since approximately 1988. Observed Data: Circumference measurements are ankles right/left 22.2/21.8cm and calves 35.5/36.0cm. Doppler evaluation of the right and left lower extremity deep venous system at the common femoral, superficial femoral, and popliteal veins demonstrates phasic spantaneaus flow with brisk augmentation. The pasterior tibial veins also have brisk augmentation present by Doppler. Duplex imaging of the right and left lower extremity deep venous systems demonstrates patent and compressible veins with no evidence of intra-luminal echogenic material and good flow by color Doppler. Duplex imaging of the right greater saphenous vein demonstrates scattered areas of echagenic material and non-compressibility in the thigh and calf region. The proximal aspect of the greater saphenous vein near the common femoral vein appears to be patent and compressible. The vascular doctor said that the impressions that he got from the evaluation with Doppler color radar was that there is no evidence or left lower extremity deep venous thrombasis. Findings are consistent with chronic superficial phlebitis of the right greater saphenous vein. These areas of the vein are likely chronically accluded. Copies of these results were sent to my family doctors office. Well I thought things could surely get better with time, because I just new in mine that there had to be a logical answer for what I was going through. A few weeks had passed, but the pains that I was having just wouldn't pass they only continued to hang around. But now there is one thing for sure, the pain would defiantly make me set down and think about a lot of things. Such as the thing called time. Because I would set and wonder how much more time it was going to take for this to be resolved it was literally getting the best of me. I couldn't sleep at night because the cramps in my legs were bad, I mean to tell you these cramps would burn and throb like crazy, but I did figure out a way to sleep a little, and that was to when I layed down, I would lay there until the pain would start up and then I would get up and walk until my legs would begin to feel cold and then I would go back to bed and lay flat on my stomach and for some odd reason I could sleep just fine. This went on for about three weeks or so, and then I noticed that suddenly it got worse. This little method that was working so good just flat quit working. I could lay down to go to sleep, and within just a few seconds I would be right back up. It's like this, the pains that I was having, was getting even worse than before, and was spreading all over my legs. When this pain would come about it would feel like my foot and leg was simply going to blow off. At this time I had an idea of what's going on. I figured that it had to be infection or a blood clot in my leg causing me these pains. But I continued to keep trying to seek some type of help. To seek help was definitely something that I had to do very soon. Because as of September 29, 1995 I had a follow-up on the thrombophlebitis. Believe it or not I had something else to show my family doctor, and that was a painful rash on my left foot something that I had dealt with for the last week or so prior to this follow-up. I intermittently had a bluish discoloration of my left great toe. My doctor said that my dorsal, pedal, and posterior tibiol pulses are good. Capillary refill was good. There was no discoloration of the foot at this time, but I had a very significant tinea infection of my great toe and lesser evidence in my other toes. I also had a wet, erosive type eruption with exudates. I also was dealing with a rash called tinea pedis according to the doctor. This was treated with miconazole cream for about two to three weeks. Between September 1995 and January 1996 I was also in and out of the doctors office.

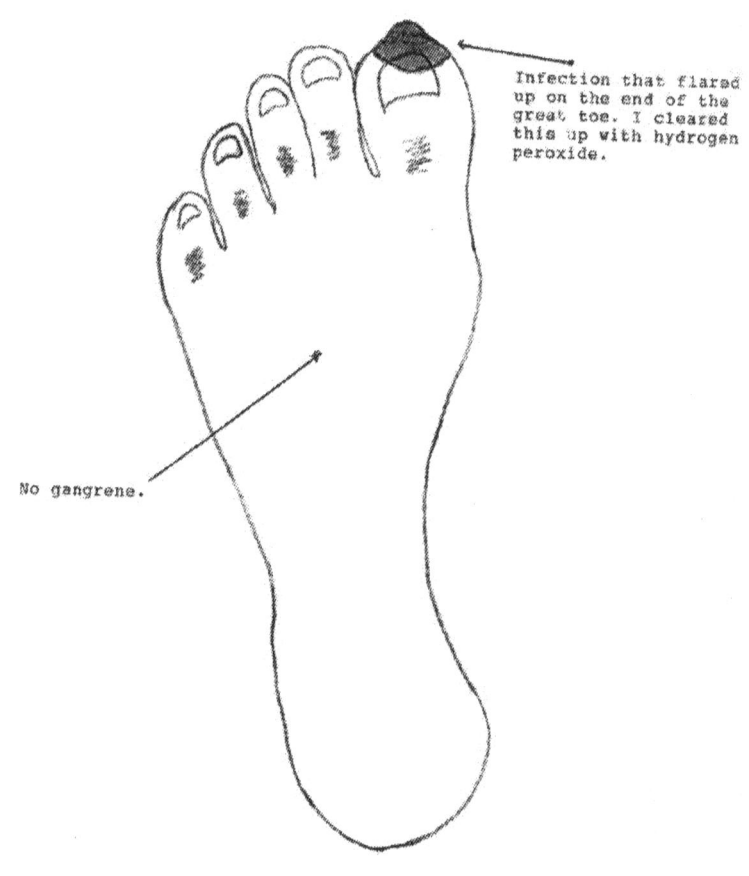

Infection that flared up on the end of the great toe. I cleared this up with hydrogen peroxide.

No gangrene.

during this time, with a head congestion. During this time the doctor said that my chest was clear, even though I had a bit of a cough which has been non-productive. The doctor said he found me to be well oriented and with no acute distress. The doctor gave me some prescriptions and told me if there was no improvement within one week that he would be glad to see me again. Well he did just that. I had returned to see the doctor on February 24, 1996, because of the fibromyalgia arthritis. I was having pains that I felt that was arthritis. Since I had received steroid injections before and it helped my symptoms, the doctor that I had to see was a step in doctor for my family doctor, and this doctor thought if this helped before when my family doctor gave me the steroid injections, it would work for me again. Guess what, it did help, but very, very little, and at this point was when I knew that I was in serious trouble and that if I didn't get serious help soon, I knew that something bad was going to happen to me. I could set down and my toes would turn blue and if I stood up and walked the color would return to my toes. What did this tell me, that I had poor circulation in my feet and this could get serious. This all means that I either have a blockage in the artery of my leg caused by infection or either I have a blockage in the artery of my leg caused by inflammation or maybe it could be a blood clot in the artery, and if this was to move down the leg, and then become to a stand still, your toes would turn blue and then it would set up an infection called gain green and then you would need a simple amputation of the left or right great toes. This could also go in the other direction and regardless if it is infection or a blood clot, it still can break loose and get to your heart or lungs and kill you during the time you are asleep or even when your awake. I was in to see the doctor on July 3, 1996 for more than what I believed to be phlebitis in my leg. Before I go any further I need to get something stated, and that is that I had been tested for "sugar" several times and it always turned out negative. I didn't have sugar trouble and still don't. Being a diabetic just didn't run in my family. When I was in to see my family doctor he said that my left foot revealed marked erythema and edma of the first three toes with what appear to be healing ulcerations in the tips of the 2nd and 3rd toes. He also said that there was good capillary refill and 1+ dorsal pedal pulses. The doctor said that there was defiantly significant cellulites present on the toes. His next step was to get me admitted to the hospital for IV antibiotics and blood test for a couple days. Well let me be the one to say, that I'm glad that I am still alive to tell the story about this painful and stressful experience that I had in my life. This all began on the third day of July 1996 when the doctor ask me to go into the hospital for a couple of days. The two days turned into a long five days, and would have probably been a lot longer if I hadn't been forced to put a stop to my time of stay. The first night of my stay in the hospital was pretty rough. The nurse had to put me an IV in my arm so that they could start some antibiotics. That wasn't the point of the matter, it was how many times it took to get the first IV to finely stop blowing out. The IV's just simply wouldn't take when the nurse would place it in the artery. It would stop up, or start leaking. As you may remember I was having trouble laying down to sleep, and the reason why was that my legs would begin to hurt me, and I would set up to sleep. Well we all know how things are when you stay in a hospital. It seems like the nurses just continue to run in and out of your room. It also seems like, the nurses do this for menus, and it also seems like when you would need the nurse for help, you may or may not get any help. Like myself, when I checked into a nearby hospital the first night was pretty rough, like I had said before. The second, third and forth nights were fair but I still can't say that they were good. What I mean by this is, that I wouldn't ask for nothing, but something for pain and that was all, and let me tell you this was out of the question. It's as simple as this, the pain that I was dealing with wasn't a joking matter. The only thing that I was getting for pain was a very small dose of Demerol from an I.V. pump. This drug wasn't effective at all, on me. I got about the same amount of relief from one aspirin a day. I finally talked the nurse into contacting my doctor, to see if I could have something a little stronger for pain. He said yes, there's no problem with that. The doctor told the nurse to give me a drug called toradol. This was a little better than before, at least this dosage of medication would ease the pain a little bit. The fifth night of my stay at the hospital really got interesting. The nurse came into my room and changed my antibiotic bag that was hooked up to my I.V. She also gave me a shot of toradol for pain, and this all took place about 6:00 o'clock that evening. I wouldn't get the pain shot again until 2:00 a.m. in the morning the nurse said. The day nurse also told my wife and I to let the night nurse know, that I was aware of the pain shot that I was going to need for pain at 2:00 a.m. Guess what, I believe I made that old girl mad. "Why", simply because I did what, anybody would have in my condition. I reminded her of my pain shot. I don't think the night nurse appreciated me doing her that way. I also think that's why she mistreated me during the last night that

I was in the hospital. What I mean when I say she mistreated me. It's very simple. She just flat out didn't bring my pain shot at 2:00 a.m. like she was supposed to. The only thing she brought to my room was "one" antibiotic bag. The nurse changed the bag out, and never at any time did she say anything about my pain shot. So when I saw that she wasn't going to say anything about it. Then I figured that I had to say something before she left my room. When I ask the nurse about the shot she just simply replied to me, real "hateful like", that she had forgot my pain shot and that she would go get it and that she would be back soon. You would never believe what I'm going to tell you. But I'm telling you the truth about this. This lady never returns to my room. I couldn't set around and wait on her all night, because I was hurting so bad that I couldn't stand it. I had decided that I should call the nurses station. I ask them where the nurse was at, and they told me that she would be there soon. Remember this all started at 2:00 a.m., and I called the nurses station at 2:30 a.m. when they told me that she would be right into my room. Well she didn't show, so I pushed the call button again and the nurses station told me that the nurse was busy and that I would just have to wait a few more minutes. I did just that, I waited. "Let's see", the clock showed 3:00 a.m. and then it showed 3:30 a.m. then 4:00 a.m. and then I had decided that I had waited long enough. I pushed the call button again, and they told me up front that they would send the nurse right in. Well this was around 4:30 when I called the nurses station, and believe it or not she finally showed up around 5:10 a.m. that morning. You would never dream of what this lady tried to pull on me. For some odd reason when the nurse came to my room to change my antibiotic bag, she never said anything about my pain shot. I just couldn't get over. The way this nurse continued to forget, my request for some type of pain reliever. It occurred to me that this woman intended to see me suffer. As I was saying before, when the nurse brought my antibiotics to my room and then turned around and told me that she forgot my pain shot. I thought to myself, for just a moment or two, about what was going on around me. That's when I began to have thoughts of getting up and just flat out telling the complete hospital staff where they could cram their big ideas of mistreatment and their little games that was played on me. To be sure that nobody gets a misunderstanding about all of this. Believe it or not the nurse finally brought in what she called pain medication for me. My opinion of what she had was a liquid form in a syringe, and this would be called "flush". Flush is a common name for a cleaner that is used to keep the I.V. cleaned and clear of plugging up. Because, if it happens to stop up the I.V. has to be changed out, and nobody likes that. The reason why I believe that the medication the nurse gave me was flush is, because when she came back to my room with what the nurse called my pain shot, she had two blue syringes, one which the nurse took off of the empty antibiotic bag that was hanging on the I.V. stand. She threw the old antibiotic bag in the garbage, and then she replaced it with a new antibiotic bag which, also had a blue syringe that was strapped on the side of it. She took both syringes out of the room with her, and she was gone for about five minutes or less, and then she returned, and it was then that the nurse finally decided to give me a dose of pain medication in my IV. She first took out the blue syringe that she said was flush, and stuck it into my IV and injected about half of the flush to clean my IV. This flush smelt like some type of alcohol or something like I had smelt before. The nurse took the remaining half of the flush that was in the blue syringe and stabbed it into the mattress beside me. Then the nurse gets out the other blue syringe, that she said was pain medicine, and began to inject it into my IV. Then the nurse attempted to do something that I would never have dreamed of or even believed, if this hadn't happened to me first hand. Before I tell yaw what the nurse tried to do. I need to get one little thing straight about something, the medicine that the nurse gave me, wasn't nothing but pure flush. It's simple, both syringes were blue, both syringes felt and smelt the same when the nurse injected them into my IV. Plus, I did not get any pain relief at all from the medicine that the nurse gave me. Now then we got that out of the way so I need to tell you what the nurse attempted to do to me. Well, believe it or not, she took the syringe out of the mattress that probably 5, to 10,000 other people plus myself had slept on, and was going to take this contaminated syringe and stick it into my IV., and try to flush it out, so that it wouldn't clot up. Let me tell you, this practice just flat out was not going to get it with my wife and me. I got out of my bed, and got fully dressed and went outside on my own will power and had a cigarette and a cup of coffee and thought everything over real good. I then went back to my room and waited until shift change time, and then my wife and I decided that we needed to bring this to somebody's attention, so we did just that, we reported this to the front office, and demanded to talk to their manager at once. It didn't seem to be a big deal to anyone at all until they realized that we were very serious about the situation and we then began to draw a crowd like you wouldn't believe. I had already been through a lot before this ever happen, so due to that my wife and I had learned a lot about doctors and hospitals and their staff and how that you are treated and mistreated in there. For example, my wife had a bad experience where she worked some time back. She has a lot of respect for elder folks and where she worked she hadn't been there long when she hired on. Her job wasn't assigned to her up front they told her that she would need to train under somebody else. She told me that the three days that she was there before she quit, that she disagreed with how the nurses staff was treating the elderly folks, and she just refused to be part of it, so she quit her job for that reason. I had several bad experiences during emergency room visits myself. SO as you can see we thought we were ready to talk and resolve the problem. But we didn't get anywhere at all, the managers showed up and we told them about what had happened and that I was in serious pain. To begin with they ordered up some type of pain killer in a syringe for me, and I new right off the bat, what that was leading up to. The nurse gave me the shot in my I.V., and then the managers proceeded to tell me that some times they would use that type of blue syringe to receive medication from containers. Then one of the managers spoke out and said that's right, and we got several colors and sizes of syringes. What was taking place here was, that they wanted it to look like the nurse was innocent of what we said she did. We thought that was pretty slick but it didn't work as planned, simply because we had our say about everything that had taken place. The doctor decided he was going to try and smooth things over by bringing in his friend which was listed a M.D., and Orthopedic doctor.

I just sit quietly while he smarted off about my illness and why that he couldn't understand why I waited so long about seeking help. I'm here to tell you, when he finished he hadn't a single idea about what my wife and I was going to say to him. I responded to his question in this manner, I told him to ask himself that question, for I have been to his office a few times for an evaluation of what he thought was causing my illness, and that he told me that I had several ruptures and a saver athletes foot infection. After that the doctor stood up and said take care of yourself and then he left the room. The next thing that the hospital tried was to worry us with things such as telling me that I better get back on some antibiotics or I could die or at least loose my foot. I must admit, I was worried, because no one knew what was causing me all this pain and torment, but yet they wouldn't let me go to see a Vascular Surgeon, and the reason why that I couldn't just get up and go on my own, was the state Tenncare coverage that I had. You are assigned to a family doctor on this coverage and you can not be treated by any other doctor than your family doctor or an Emergency room, with out your family doctors written consent. The only way that you could go out and see another doctor would be with cash money and that would have to take place out of state because in the state of Tennessee if you were on the Tenncare program and you set out to seek a doctor on your own they wouldn't be aloud to except cash payment from you, if you lived in the state of Tennessee nor could another doctor treat you without a referral from your family doctor. If this took place at anytime the state could come down hard on these doctors if it was found out, because the state has a signed contract with the clinical doctors and hospitals. So as you can see what my wife and I were up against, this was only the beginning of all the headaches and aggravation. Anyway I was taken to get X-rays and my family doctor decided that he would try to get my wife to tell him about what the nurse had did that night to me. When I was returned to my room my wife told me about what just took place, and she also told me that she agreed with me, that I needed to get out of that hospital because everyone was sticking together they would handle this in a suitable way, and that this would definitely be brought to the nurses attention. The wife and I knew in our minds that nothing would be done about the malpractice that took place during my last night of stay in the hospital. My doctor tried to get me to stay in the hospital a little longer, but I knew I couldn't, because I felt like I needed to be seen by a Vascular doctor, and somehow I had to figure out a way to do so. So I ask my wife to gather my things, and I signed myself out of the hospital and we went home. The following day my family doctor had his nurse to try and talk me in to coming in for a visit so he could get me set up to go see a Vascular specialist he said. My wife and I fell for the story and we went to my family doctors office and boy, was that a bad move. The only thing that we got there was criticizing of why I left the hospital and why I wouldn't get back in the hospital. I finally decided that my wife and I had took enough of this, so cut this little meeting short. My wife was upset about the situation after our doctor said he rather we found ourselves a new family doctor. I brought it to his attention about the state tenncare law and that I was very aware of how it works. See it's like this just about anywhere. Your family doctor is supposed to give you a notice. The question here is, can a doctor ever dismiss a patient? Yes. But the doctor must take extreme care so that he or she isn't charged with abandonment. Listen! Once the doctor establishes a patient doctor relationship, a contract exists and the doctor has consented to provide treatment and care for the patient. The doctor may wish to dismiss a patient because the patient won't agree to co-operate with the treatment plans or fails to keep appointments. Sometimes, too, it's necessary for the doctor to dismiss a patient when the doctor retires, relocates, or discontinues to practice medicine for any other reason. If any of these situations arise, it's necessary for the doctor to do a number of things: The doctor must give notice to the patient within 14 days or more of dismissal. Second, the doctor must send a dismiss letter to the patient which includes the date, the reason for dismissal or assist on the transfer of records, and the doctors signature. A copy of the letter must be placed in the patients medical records. The doctor also must address the letter to the patient or guardian. Next the doctor must send the letter by certified mail and request a return receipt. The doctor also must place a copy of the signed receipt in the patients medical records. This type of dismissal procedure doesn't apply to a patient in a hospital, however, a hospital can't terminate treatment once it has been initiated. Well to the best of my knowledge I've never received nothing like this. I was out hangen in the wind. My doctor said that if I would go back into their hospital that he would continue being my family doctor. I didn't fall for that old trick, to be honest I came out of the hospital worse off than I was when I went in. So after a few days past, I soon realized that I didn't have a family doctor, so I just decided to set out on my own and find a doctor that could tell me what was causing me to have all these illnesses problems I guess its safe to say that I had a gut feeling that my time here on God's green earth was coming to a end, and very fast. You would never believe me if I said that I could feel, smell, and taste death not to far down the road, when I checked out of the hospital, but I was determined to go out fighting. There wasn't a single person that believed in what I had to say but my wife and son. At this point I don't believe that my family or friends outside my wife and my little boy, believed that I was really as sick as my wife and I said I was. I've pushed my self to the limit several times even though the pains that I was having was really bad. I would get out and cut the grass I would go a little ways and my legs would lock up tight on me, and I couldn't walk no more, and I would set down and begin to rub my legs because it felt like everything in my legs had been pulled out. Seemed like the pain would never leave my legs and it also took several minutes for the feeling to return to my legs, but I would get up and go at it again. A little more time had past by, and things had got a little worse and I had seen several other doctors. Lets see now, between two states I had been talked to or treated by about five emergency room doctors and about twenty eight clinical M.D., doctors. A lot of these doctors were very good at there jobs but nobody could tell me something that I didn't already know. I recall of one emergency room doctor that treated my wife and I, like we were pure trash, and that we were taking up his time. I had been to a couple of Orthopedic doctors the first one said that he thinks that the hernias I have is my problems. The other one said that he believed it was caused by fibromyalgia arthritis, that was in my nerves system, I also went to a Baptist pain center.

*A True Story of Misdiagnosed/Unexplainable Pains
Found to be Caused by Tobacco Use*

They also believed that the problem was in my nerves system. I had been observed by a cardiovascular surgeon, and he believed that the circulation in my legs was very poor. But he also stated that he could not treat me, for this wasn't his trade in the medical field, so he referred me to a rheumatolagy specialist in hopes that I would receive some type of help. Well I did and I didn't get any help from the rheumatologist, he gave me a prescription for the pain and a small prescription for antibiotics and he ask that I come to his office and clinic that was about sixty five miles on up the road, because he would like to get a second opinion on me. So in a few weeks my brother took my wife and I up to this clinic, where the rheumatologist ask that I come to. Well the second opinion come from a internal medicine physician that worked at this clinic. His findings was a chronic foot infection and felt that I should continue to be treated with antibiotics and other measures that might lead up to surgery for "aortoiliac by pass". There was some talk about an arteriogram for me but this never took place. The doctor felt that I was

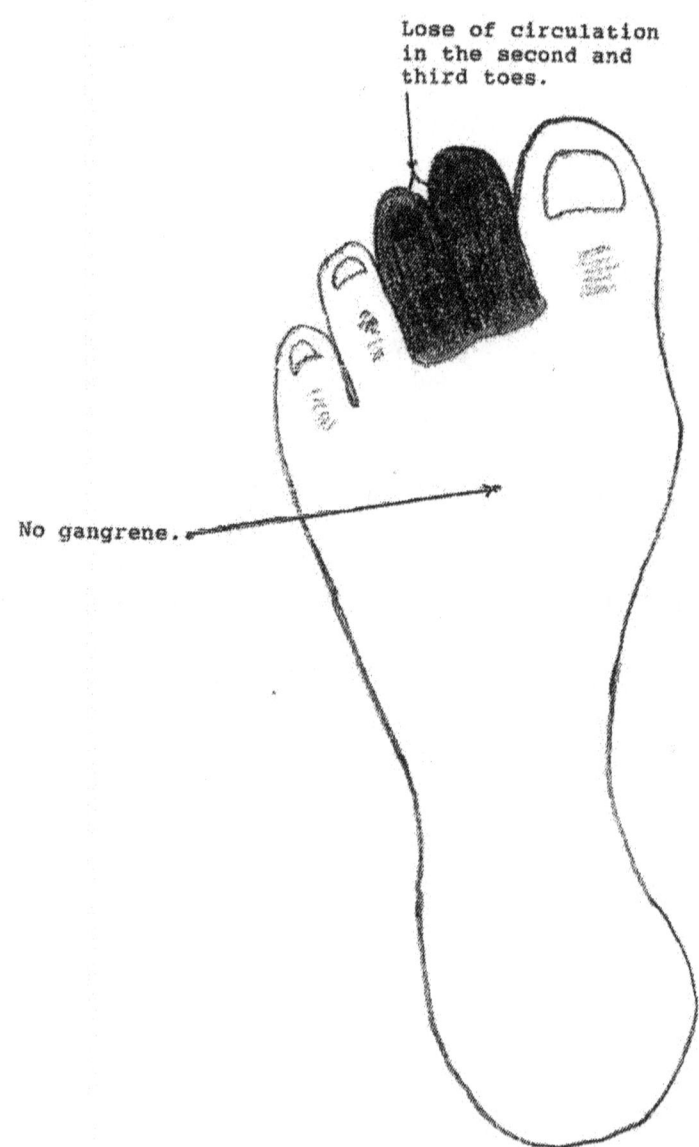

Lose of circulation
in the second and
third toes.

No gangrene.

having some type of allergic reaction linked to my cigarette smoking., during this visit I had with the Internal Medicine Physician, and he advised me that it would be at my best interest to quit smoking as soon as possible. But I just continued on to smoke cigarettes, simply because it seemed to calm my nerves down, and my nerves was definitely on the edge at this time. Well this last doctors appointment took place on September 17, 1996 and it was my last one for a while, because I just flat out quit going. I simply felt like it was a waste of time, because every doctor I went to either pushed me away or just simply had me to keep coming back and the wildest thing was that I was the one to suffer when everything was said and done for. For the month's of October, November and December was truly nothing but pure misery, for me and my family. By the first week of October I was no longer able to do anything much at all other than set around and grieve and look out the windows and wish that the pain in my legs and foot would come to a end, and that my health would get better. By the middle of October I had to use crutches to get around and if I didn't, I simply couldn't get up and walk, and go anywhere. I was in bad shape as far as my health goes, and I knew that I couldn't bring an income in to our home anymore and I needed my family's support. My wife and little boy was there for me every step of the way. My wife got us some help along the way, from my parents and hers, but that was just about it.

It was like, if no one believed that my condition was really that bad. About the only thing that I did try to do, during these past three months, was to take and really push myself to go about 60 miles down the road from my home, to hear a judge that worked for the Social Security Office, talk to my wife and I as if he felt that we were worthless to the human society. That didn't go over so good with my lawyer, so he reminded the judge of what we were there for, and that was to see if the judge felt that I was eligible for Social Security Disability Income. The answer that we needed from the judge, come very quickly. We revealed this by the way the judge handled his words and his tone of voice when he would talk to my lawyer, my wife and myself about the situation. But, now let me get one thing straight first. My decision for Social Security Disability didn't come through until about one year and a half later. It was just as we figured it would be. My Social Security Disability decision was unfavorable to me. This decision was made by the reciting judge over my case, and then a registered letter was sent out to me by mail to let me know what the decision was. Before I leave this subject I would like to say that if I could have gotten my health back up to par, I would have never signed up for Social Security Disability because of all the trouble and pain that my wife and I were put through, during the two and a half years trying to get a decision from the Social Security Administration. I had trouble with finding a doctor to back me up on my health problems. "Stop and think about this for a few minutes", I had been treated by 32 doctors, and I had visited 5 emergency rooms during this time, and was sent to 3 Social Security doctors so that they could give there opinions to the State Social Security Board of their findings, when they gave me a health physical. But nobody wanted to step up and say that I was unable to work. Every doctor had the same answer for my lawyer and the Social Security Board. The patient is being treated for a lot of different things, but I can't answer that question because I don't know if he can work or not. At this time I was being treated for Arthritis, Phlebitis of the vein, skin rashes, back trouble, hernias, you name it and it seemed like I was being treated for it. But still nobody would back me up and say that I was unable to work 8 to 10 hours a day on a public job. I knew in my mind that I absolutely could not hold down a public job at this time, I was in to much pain and my nerves was very, very high. Check out all the medications that I was on or had taken already. Amoxicillin 500 MG caps, Acetaminophen #3, Nizoral, Lorazepam 1 MG, Ibuprofen 800 MG, Zantac 150 MG Tabs, Cyclobenzaprine 10 MG, Imipramine 50 MG, Pen-Vee K 500Mg Tabs, Amitriptyline 25 MG, Paxil 20 MG-okky, Amitriptyline 50MG, Ibuprofen 600 MG, Cimetidine 400MG, Paxil 20 MG, Amitriptyline 50MG, Paxil 20MG, Ibuprofen 600 MG Mapap 500MG, Cimetidine 400MG, Amitriptyline 50 MG, Mapap 500MG, Cimetidine 400MG, Ibuprofen 600MG, Mapap 500MG, Ibuprofen 600MG, Amitriptyline 50MG, Cimetidine 800MG, Diphenhydramine 25MG, Miconazole cream, Trazodone 100MG, Acetaminophen #3, Trazodone 100MG, Hydroxyzine HCL, trazodone 100MG, Miccoazole Cream 15MG, Cyclobenzaprine 10MG, Doxepin 25MG, Cephalexin 500MG, Ibuprofen 600MG, Cimetidine 800MG, Vancenase AQ, Diphenhydramine 25MG, Amoxicillin 500MG, Cephalexin 500MG, Cimetidine 400MG, Lortab 7.5MG, Cephalexin 500MG, Vicodine Tabs, Restoril 30MG, Prednisone 10MG, Cephalexin 500MG, Lortab 7.5MG, Cephalexin 500MG, Percocet, Vicodine Tabs, Prednisone 10MG, Cephalexin 500MG, Vicodin tabs Cephalexin 500MG, Percocet, Coumadin 5MG, Augmentin 250MG, Bactroban, Acetaminophen #3,

Indomethacin 50MG, Augmentin 250MG, Prednisone 10MG, Percocet, Lortab 7.5MG, Augmentin 500MG, Coumadin 5MG, Acetaminophen #3. Over the past three years "all of this medication," but yet nobody thinks or agrees that I was disabled and unable to work on a public job 8 to 10 hours a day, regardless of what anybody thought, the judge said he felt that I could work on a public job, even if it meant that I had to stand or set all day. I finally just gave up on the doctors and the Social Security Office all together. At this point, as far as a doctor goes, I didn't have one. I was pretty much on my own, so I had

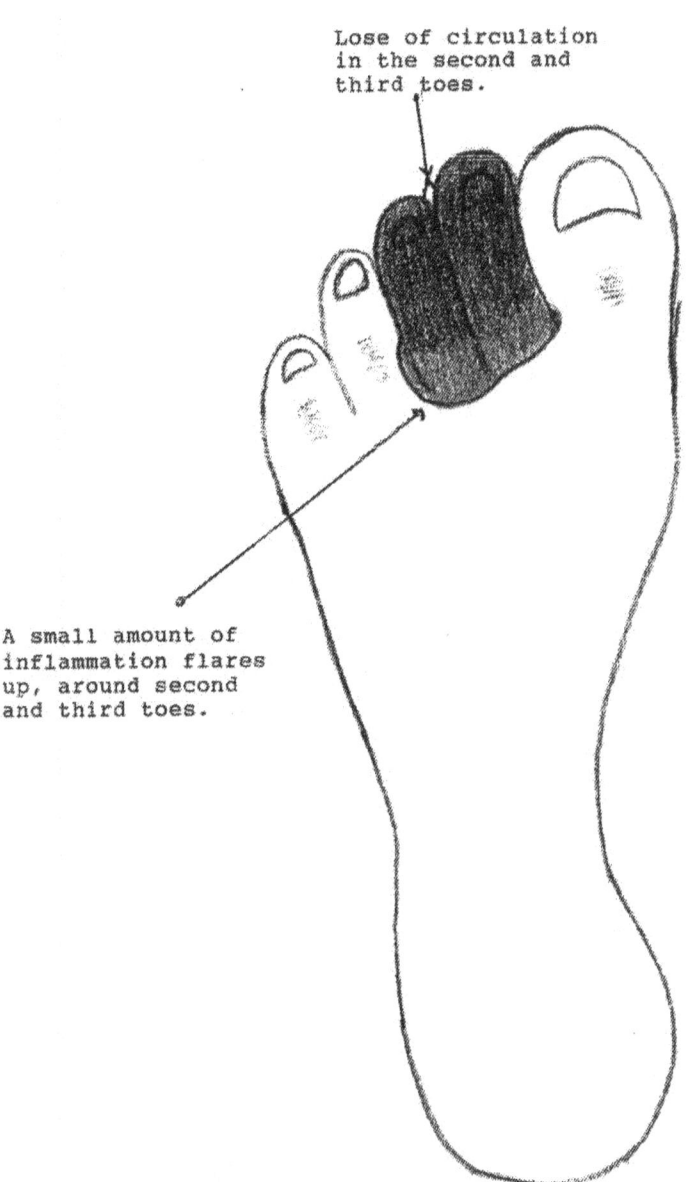

Lose of circulation
in the second and
third toes.

A small amount of
inflammation flares
up, around second
and third toes.

to begin to doctor myself. I found that I could use Neosporin with pain reliever in it, to coat my toes. Due to the gangrene that was on my foot and toes, I had to deal with a lot of pain and burning. I would put the Neosporin all over my foot and toes and it seemed to ease the pain, plus it would build a thick hard crust over the gangrene so that the air couldn't hit it, and cause it to burn bad. I would send my wife to get something new every day, to try out on my foot to see if I could get it to begin to heal a little more, and to ease the pain a little more to. I had so much infection built up in my body, that I would have what felt like electrical shocks to come through my teeth at times, and im telling you it felt like the top of my head was going to blow off. But the wife and I, just continued on trying different things. My wife could probably be a trainee doctor after all she had went through with me during this time. There was a lot of different things took place during the middle to the last of October.

Things like my foot had gotten worse and I had to give up the crutches as far as getting around. My wife had to go out and find me a wheel chair, because it had got to the point that I couldn't stand my leg and foot to be in the downward position when I would be standing up, so as you see, I could set in the wheel chair and prop up my bad foot and leg and still I could get around through the house to do the things that I needed to do. I really was excited when the wife brought in the wheelchair because, I could finally get off the couch or out of the bed and go outside on the porch and get some fresh air and to be able to watch my wife and little boy play ball or ride the four wheeler. Even though I had the privilege to get out on the porch, that didn't mean that I was worry free, and pain free. As I would watch my wife and little boy do things together, it would still bother me. I had got to the point to where I would grieve and cry inside because I had realized that my little boy was growing up, and I couldn't enjoy the most precious time of his life, but the wife and I just continued to hope and pray that things would get better. Even though this wasn't a easy task for my wife. She would take care of me, and try to make time to play with our little boy, and give him the attention that all little kids need. I tried to do a lot of things myself, but there were some things that, I was just flat out not able to do myself. My wife said that I amazed her, with the things that I could do, during the time that I was down with my legs and foot. I had learned to do a lot of things on my own because of the countless nights, that I would set around in my wheelchair, because I literally could not lay down and sleep, because of the pain that I was having in my legs and foot. Trust me, if there was any possible way that this guy could have slept I would have. I know it don't sound logical, for any one human to make it on 30 minutes sleep every 24 hours, but I am here to tell you that I did, and definitely not by choice. My wife had ask me this same question so many times, that I couldn't count them all. And that was, is there something that she could do for me, to help ease the pain a little, and all that I could say was, no there's not. Bless her heart, she wanted to and tried to help me anytime that I would ask her to. It took me forever to convince my wife to try and lay down and get some sleep at night. But she was worried that I might need something. We finally come to an agreement to what would be the best for the both of us, and our little boy. And that was that I all ready had enough pain to kill anything alive seemed like, and that if I needed her for something that I would definitely wake her up from sleep and tell her what I was needing or if something was bad wrong. It was every 20 to 30 minutes that she was checking on me. I would set in the bathroom in tears and in a lot of pain, with the door shut so that I wouldn't wake up my family. But it seemed like my wife had ears like a hawk, as the old saying goes. She would be at my side in a matter of seconds, if she heard as much as a little whimper from me. But you know something, I tried to be quiet but it was just impossible, because of the pain that I was having, was so bad. I was taking pain killers for the pain, but it wasn't helping to ease the pain, because of what I believed to be a blockage in the deep artery in the left leg. I got more relief by wearing an ace bandage around the leg and foot for some reason, and I think this was caused by slowing down the blood flow in the artery, and when the blood would reach the blockage in the artery it would have enough time to flow through the blockage without pooling up. What I mean by pooling up is, that if you try to poor a gallon of water through something, like a oil funnel that has a hole in it, about the size of a pencil. We all know what would happen here. The water would just back up and run over. Well there you have it, that's what I think was going on with my leg and foot. Due to the blockage, the blood would back up in the deep artery of my leg and begin to clot up itself, if I hadn't kept using the ace bandages on my leg and foot. Speaking of ace bandages, there several other devices that I had to wear to. Such as wrist bands that were special made for sprains and arthritis. I also had to wear a back brace for the back spasms. I had to wear a truss for what the doctor called irritated ruptures. I also had to wear men's support hose to help the circulation in my legs. To tell the truth, by the time I got all these devices on I felt like a mummy walking around. I knew that I couldn't go on like this so my wife began to surf through the phone book, to try to find me help once again. We did this for a couple of days, until we found a doctor that would at least try to help. Around October 22, 1996 the wife and I was still in search for some type of help or at least some answers to what was causing all of these really bad pains in my legs and foot. So we decided to call up a certain kind of foot doctor. This foot doctor, claimed that he could treat Athletes foot and poison of the foot, so I told the wife that I couldn't loose nothing in the deal and she agreed. So I got a appointment set up for that afternoon with this doctor. I have to say this much right off the bat. I was pleased with how this doctor spoke to me. He spoke to the wife and I like he was concerned about my foot first, and appreciated our business second. This guy didn't waste no time, he went right to work. With my permission he did a local block. These 4 shots of buffered Lidocaine, numbed the foot a little but not completely. After he did this local block he did some debrigement of the two toes. What debrigement on my behalf, was to pull the dead gangrene skin off of my toes. After he finished I had to take a few deep breaths of air, because by then the nerve was uncovered, and didn't seem like there was anything that would stop the pain then, for sure. But this old boy was going to try one way or another to help me, and I greatly appreciated every thing this doctor was doing even if it turned out to be wrong. This wasn't a easy task for this doctor to heal, because I had the two toes that was blue and black with dry gangrene about three quarter the way covered over the toes. As if that wasn't enough, I had wet gangrene all over the top of my foot, and it was about to drive me out of my mind. It would itch to the bone for about 15 minutes, and then all of a sudden it would start burning like fire. The foot doctor thought maybe that I had some possible allergic reaction to the Neosporin, so he decided

A True Story of Misdiagnosed/Unexplainable Pains
Found to be Caused by Tobacco Use

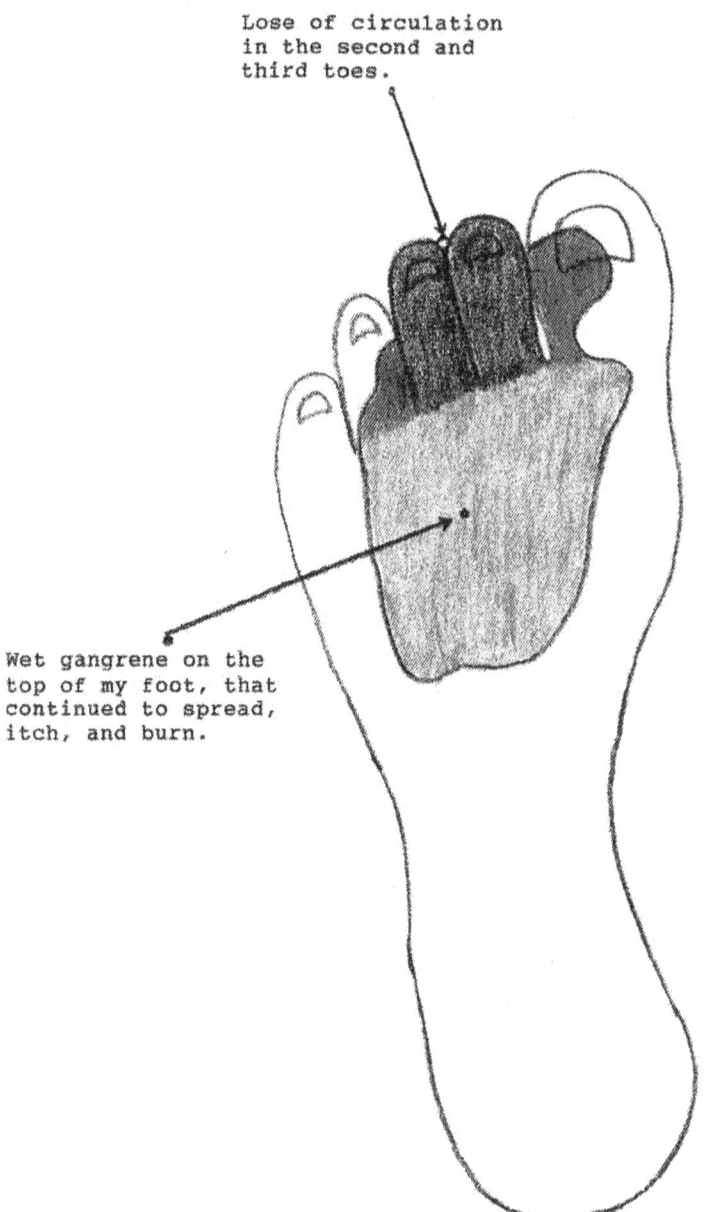

Lose of circulation
in the second and
third toes.

Wet gangrene on the
top of my foot, that
continued to spread,
itch, and burn.

to try an ointment called Bactraban. He dressed the top of my foot down with the Bactroban and rapped it up with white gauze bandage. The doctor also placed me on Vicodin to ease the pain and Restoril 30mg at night to help me sleep. I told the doctor that I had taken the pain killer called Percocet, and it didn't seem to help much at all. The doctor said that he could also try to block the dorsal cutaneous nerve, the deep peroneal, and the sapheneous nerve to the left foot with Lidocaine and Marcaine mixture to give me a few hours of relief, so that I could get some sleep. Even though it was going to hurt like crazy I told the doctor to go for it. The doctor was right, it gave me about four hours of relief, even though it didn't completely numb the pain in my foot. By the time I got home, two hours had passed by, but I did get about two hours of sleep with my leg hanging off the side of the bed, because I couldn't lay down flat on the bed, regardless whether it was numbed or not. The doctor also gave me a prescription for Augmentin 250mg, Twice daily for two weeks., and a prescription for tapering Prednisone. The Prednisone was to be taken completely up in seven days. The first day I would need to take seven tablets, the second day six, the third day five, the fourth day four, the fifth day three, the sixth day two, the seventh day one., so as you can see, it would be all gone by the seventh day. The foot doctor said that he would like to see me back in his office in two weeks. This was two weeks of my life that I will never forget. The first day after taking the Prednisone wasn't to bad. But the second day was a total different deal. My foot was itching and burning at the same time, on top of my foot, where the wet gangrene was located. Every day that went by, I noticed that the itching was leaving, and the burning was increasing by the last day, that I was to take the prednisone, I realized what was causing this burn, and that was the Prednisone. I had one tablet left to take, so I went ahead and took it because I figured if this medication was going to help me, I was going to suffer for a few days. The burning was pretty bad that first week, but I was able to keep ice packs on the burn and I could live with it. There was no comparison, to the burn from the first week to the second week. By the first week of November 1996 I was literally going crazy mad., I was loosing my mind. To be honest about it, I was as suicidal as they get. I'm going to tell you just exactly what this burn felt like. Take your bare foot and set it down into a pit of red hot, coal clinkers. I'm telling you something that is the truth. I had a burn before, that was said to be a first degree burn on my hand, I could pack it in ice and get a little relief. But this burn that I had on my foot was a evil burn. It was burning so bad one night I went out on my front porch with out any coverage at all on my foot, and it was flat pouring the ice and snow. The wind was so cold that you absolutely, could freeze to death, if you didn't have a lot of winter clothing on. I had my wife to fix me up two really good ice packs. She brought them to me, and I wrapped my foot up with them, and then I put myself two coats on and wrapped the blanket around me, that the wife had brought me also.

Well! There I set, as if I didn't have a brain one, as the old saying goes. But it's as simple as this I had to try something fast, because this burn was just like I said it was. It was a evil burn. I set there until the ice packs had turn my foot completely blue and purple, and it just continued right on burning just like nobodies business, I'm telling you. It was like a bad nightmare, and I couldn't wake up from it. I tried several types of burn ointments, and it just seemed like nothing would work at all. I believe I tried every old remedy that I could think of or had heard of to try and cool off the

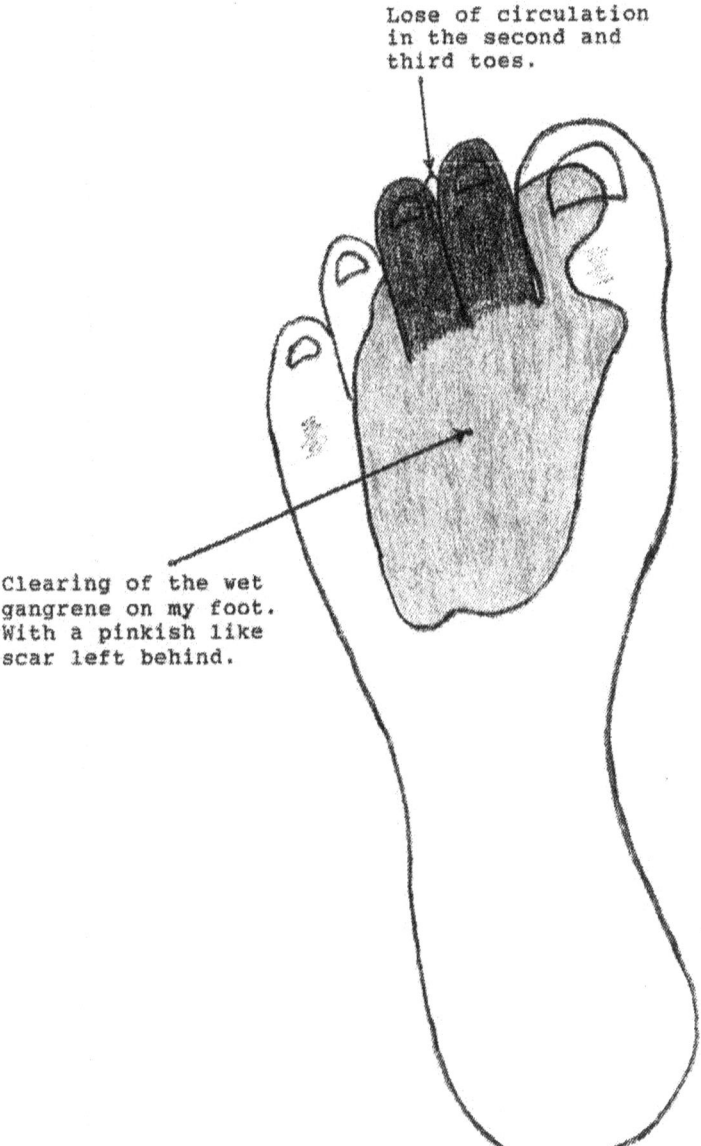

A True Story of Misdiagnosed/Unexplainable Pains
Found to be Caused by Tobacco Use

Lose of circulation
in the second and
third toes.

Clearing of the wet
gangrene on my foot.
With a pinkish like
scar left behind.

burning on my foot. But nothing would faze it. That's when I new for sure that I was going to lose "my life" if something good didn't happen for me very soon. When someone tells you that there dying or they can feel, smell, or taste death, you better try to take a little time and listen to them for a change. Because it could easily be your husband, wife, brother, sister, your child or friend and they may be a chance that they know there dying. It wasn't only the burning that made me feel and think this. I new that my blood was contaminated with infection and this could damage my heart. Also it was very possible that the gangrene could have gotten into my blood stream, and that could cause a lot of damage, maybe even death. I will say this much, I wouldn't wish the pain and burning that I've gone through on my worst enemy. That's what I told my foot doctor when I had to go for a follow up on my foot. This follow up I believe was on or around November 2, 1996. The doctor did a little more debridgement of the toes of the second and third toes. Then he cleaned and redressed my foot, and wrapped it up with gauze. He also apologized to me, for the really bad burning reaction that I had with the prednisone tablets that I was taking. But also never failed to let me know that it was for my best interest. The doctor was definitely right about this, because the wet gangrene had almost cleared up, on the top of my foot. During this last visit with the doctor he said that my foot was coming along nicely, and that he would like to see me back in his office in about three weeks. I did what the doctor told me to, and that was to continue to take all of my medications, as directed. The medications that the doctor prescribed to me, was the same as the last time, but he didn't prescribe the prednisone again, because he said that

70

it wasn't good to take it for long periods of time. Because of the side effects that it has. The doctor had set me up an appointment to come in on or around November 22, 1996. When I went to this appointment, the foot doctor said that he was pleased to see the wet gangrene was gone, and that the foot was coming along nicely. The doctor also did a little more debrigement on my toes, and said that he would like to keep me on the medication a little while longer if possible, and that he would see me again in about two more weeks. That would have been around, December 12, 1996. So I suffered for three more weeks with pain in my foot and toes. I couldn't even sleep, days or nights, it didn't matter. I was taking a lot of morphine and a lot of high potent anti-depressants and I would still be setting up looking around. The only thing that I could figure, was the medicine couldn't reach the pain in my toes, because I had a blockage in my leg and foot preventing it to do so. Well the next three weeks had finally past, and I was glad, because the pain in my foot had me going nuts, and I was ready to try something new on my foot. So when I went for my next appointment I had decided that I was going to ask the doctor if he could give me a cortisone shot in my foot for the pain. I had a idea of what might happen if the cortisone was injected into the toe area where the two toes were infected and had the gangrene set up on them. I had heard that if you try to inject cortisone into a area where there is infection that it would kill the tissue in the area. Well the doctor said that he would rather not do that, but I wouldn't stop at that. I told him that if he would do this, that I would sign whatever papers that it took. He ask me first, before he injected the cortisone into my foot, why do you insist on doing this. I told him this. I've had cortisone shots before, for arthritis pains, and it would put the stop on the pain. But I also new that arthritis was caused by inflammation, not by infection. I also didn't have nothing to lose, because half of each toe, is already dead. The doctor went ahead with the cortisone injection in my foot. There was a little catch to this. The needle had to enter just below the ankle and go through the tissue or muscle until it reached the two toes that had begun to turn black. Please see pitcher numbered as "6A".

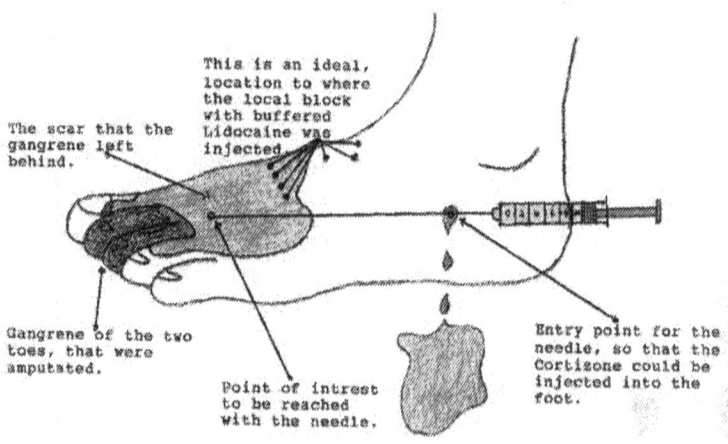

This is an ideal, location to where the local block with buffered Lidocaine was injected.

The scar that the gangrene left behind.

Gangrene of the two toes, that were amputated.

Point of intrest to be reached with the needle.

Entry point for the needle, so that the Cortizone could be injected into the foot.

I often wondered how I was able to set and take the shot of cortisone into my foot. The reason why that I say this is, because my foot was still swelled really bad with infection, and the doctor entered the needle into my foot just below the ankle and pushed the long needle all the way through to my second and third toes. This was very painful, due to the infection and inflammation in my foot. I could literally feel the tissue tearing as the needle was sliding through my foot. After the doctor injected the cortisone into my foot, he dragged the needle back out of my foot, and the blood literally poured. The bleeding didn't want to stop, so the doctor rapped my foot up in gauze for a little while, until it did stop bleeding. Then the doctor cleaned my foot up again, and dressed the two toes and the top of my foot with an antibiotic cream and rapped it up with a fresh roll of gauze. The doctor gave me a refill on my medicines and told me that he would like to see again in about two weeks. I believe there was about four days that had past by, and I had to call up the foot doctor and break the bad news, and that was to tell him that both of my toes were completely black. Both the second and third toes were dead. The foot doctor told me that if the two toes have turned completely black, there was nothing more that he could do for me, other than recommend me to a Vascular Surgeon. I ask the foot doctor, if it was possible that he could refer me to a Vascular Surgeon, because of the type of insurance that I had. He said that he could do this for me, with in a few minutes. Sure enough he did just what he said he could do. He called me back in just a few minutes and told me that he had got in touch with the Vascular Surgeons office, and that they agreed to see me later that day on an emergency bases. My appointment was scheduled for December 16, 1996 at 4:30 in the evening, with the Vascular Surgeons. When the wife and I reached the Vascular Surgeons office, they took me right on in, and I didn't have to wait at all. These doctors handled themselves very professionally, I noticed. The chief Vascular surgeon began to examine me. The doctor said according to my medial records, that the foot doctor had sent over to him, that I apparently had problems with migratory thrombophlebitis in the legs for approximately five or six years. In fact, the doctor found where I had stated to the foot doctor that in 1987 I developed superficial phlebitis and slowing of the legs. The doctor also found that I had been in there office in July 1995 to see one of there doctors. However, the doctor at this time did not find a deep venous thromboisis and recommended that I take an aspirin a day for chronic superficial phlebitis of the right greater sophenous vein. These veins he said, appeared to be chronically occluded. The doctor ask me if I was a smoker still, and I said no. I was told that I needed to try and quit smoking that it may be a lot of my problems. I decided I would try to quit, so I started on chewing tobacco, to get my mind off of smoking. I was sent to the Vascular laboratory the same day of my first visit, and found to have equal blood pressure in both arms and normal thigh, calf, and ankle pressures. However, I had severe small vessel disease with TBI of 0.31 on the right great toe and no audible flow in the left great toe. The doctor also said there was no evidence of any aortic or ilioc disease. There appears to be severe small vessel disease in the left foot. I revealed to the vascular surgeon that I had a history of arthritis, asthma, superficial migratory thrombophlebitis, heart burn, peptic ulcer disease, and I believed that I was a "free bleeder". I also told the vascular surgeon that the most recent medication I had was percocet, augmentin, and tapering dose of prednisone. The vascular surgeon said that my blood pressure was 140/80, temperature 96. Lungs! Clear to ausculation and percussion, Heart: Regular rhythm with no murmur. Abdomen: Scaphoid, soft. The doctor said that I had excellent bilateral femoral pulses as well as excellent popliteal pulses, but had no pedal pulses that he could feel. He also said that I had erythema of both feet, but much worse on the left. What this means, is redness of the skin due to congestion of the capillaries. The doctor revealed to me that the left foot appears to also have cellulites of the distal foot, including all the toe's on the left foot. Before I move on, let me explain what cellulites is. It is inflammation of the soft or connective tissue, in which a thin, watery exudates spreads through the clevage plans of interstitial and tissue spaces; it may lead to ulceration and abscess. I also had dry gangrene of the second and third toes, which I stated to the doctor that they had become much worse over the last two or three days. The doctor said that it looks to him like I've got, 1. Severe arterio-sclerotic occlusive disease of the left lower extremity with gangrene of the second and third toes. 2. Cellulitis of the left foot. 3. Probable bilateral small vessel disease in the toes of both feet. 4. History of peptic ulcer disease. 5. Arthritis. 6. Asthma. 7. Migratory thrombo-phlebitis. 8. Reflux esophagitis. 9. History of being "a free bleeder", due to all of the ibuprofen and coumadin that I had taken in the past. 10. Still had a tobacco addiction. After the doctor finished his examination of me, I ask him what his recommendation for me was. He answered my question very quickly. He said that he felt that I need to be admitted into the hospital on an emergency basis for intensive IV antibiotics. Also need to have an arteriogram with attention to the pedal arch and digital vessels. The doctor also revealed that I need to have detailed care of the left foot with antibiotic dressings, and application of Nitroglycerin paste to the foot. The Vascular surgeon also told me that I must not use tobacco of any sort and that most likely I would lose at least the two toes and possible the distal foot or left leg and that if I continued to smoke I would most likely be a bilateral amputee within five to ten years. Here are the results of the, Lower Extremity Arterial Evaluation.

Location	Pressure RT	Pressure LT	Indices RT	Indices LT
Brachial	130	130		
Thigh	140	150		
Calf	130	120		
PTA	118	102	0.91	0.78
ATA	122	110	0.94	0.85
Great Toe	40	0	0.31	0

This study was difficult as I could only lie down for a minimal amount of time. However, the tech was able to interrogate into visualize what I understood to be the common femoral, profundus femoral, superficial femoral, popliteol, and the tibiol vessels. Most folks may not understand what all these numbers and words mean, but this is the most interesting part of this story. What this all means is, that there was a little blood circulation in the right leg, and little to none in the left leg. I didn't have a clue of what any of this meant, until I got down sick and unable to walk. It was then that I took an interest in reading health books of any kind. If I could find a health book that had something in it that even sounded like the problems that I was having I would pick it up and take to reading it. So there you have it, that's how I was able to understand a little bit about these test and there purpose. Here is some more results from the Arterial Evaluation. The bronchial blood pressure was 130mm hg bilaterally. The thigh, calf, and ankle levels were equal bilaterally with an ankle/brachial index of 0.94 in the right ankle and 0.85 on the left. Toe/brachial index was 0.31 in the right great toe and there wasn't no flow at all that could be detected on the left great toe by PPG. Imaging of the large vessels from common femoral down through the mid calf level revealed no evidence of flow reducing plaque. Doppler wave forms were triphasic down through the popliteal level bilaterally. The anterior and posterior tibial Doppler examination at the ankle revealed, what the tech called monophasic wave forms with marked turbulence. PPG of the toes were nearly flatline with the exception of the left fifth toe. The impression that the Vascular surgeon got from the Doppler and pressure test, revealed that I had a very severe small vessel disease much worse on the left than the right. The Vascular doctor also said that the findings were compatible with the gangrene of the second and third toes on my left foot. You know something, during the time that these test were taking place I would weary about what the next test would be like, and I would wonder if it was going to hurt or not. I had just got to the point to where I couldn't take pain anymore. I ask the tech that was doing all of these test, if there was going to be any test that would inflict a lot of pain to me, and he said not that I'm aware of he said. There was also a chest exam performed. The heart was normal in size and contour. The lungs were well expanded and clear. The chest exam finished out the day, and I was really glad because, I was ready to get placed into my room in the hospital, so that I could begin receiving treatments for the pain in my foot and leg. Well as you can remember, I was admitted into the hospital on December 16, 1997 at 9:00 o'clock p.m. in the late afternoon. When I reached my room, I was told that I wasn't allowed to smoke, regardless of how bad I was craving a cigarette. As a cigarette smoker, you could imagine what was going through my head. I set and thought to myself for just a few minutes, and then I ask myself if I could do without the cigarettes, or do I continue to smoke and put myself at more of a risk of having to have my complete leg amputated. Well I chose to try and not smoke. I will admit I got to the point , to where I didn't think I was going to be able to give up the cigarettes, but I did survive, especially after the nurse put a IV in my arm, and then he turned around and gave me a injection of valium I believe it was, and I can easily say it just flat out put me in another world, but It didn't seem to ease the pain at all. That first night in the hospital, was a proven fact of what I told the doctors, I would do for sleep at home. After the nurse gave me the shot of valium or whatever it was, I was on a serious high, but I also was very sleepy to. I tried to lay down on the bed and sleep but I couldn't, because my foot felt like it was going to blow off at any time. I'm telling you, I was in some serious pain. That first night I got a little sleep, and did this by being drugged up and sleeping on my wife's shoulder while she held me up right, simply because I couldn't lay down and sleep. Now wasn't that really nice of my wife to do this for me, I think so. Well the following day was already set up for me. I was scheduled to get an arteriogram. This was on December 17, 1997. The doctors had already talked to me, about the risks and the benefits of the procedure of the arteriogram the night before the test was performed, and the doctor also gave the wife and I a sheet of paper with all the information that we would want to know about how the arteriogram works. The information sheet that was given to the wife and I would read as follows.

PURPOSE: An angiogram is an x-ray that lets your doctors look inside your arteries to help discover blockages or narrowings, or other changes in your blood vessels. An injected "dye" outlines the arteries and highlights the problems. Changes in your arteries can affect any of the organs in your body. As soon as the angiogram pinpoints the problem, your doctors can choose the best treatment for it.

PREPARATION: This test may be done on an outpatient basis or you may check into the hospital the day before. Do not eat or drink anything, take your medicine with a few sips of water but check with your nurse or doctor first. Before the angiogram, you will put on a hospital gown. You can keep your dentures in and glasses on during the test. Just before you go to the x-ray room you will be asked to urinate to empty your bladder. A nurse will put an intravenous (IV) needle into a vein in your arm. The IV will be used to give you fluids and medicines during the angiogram. Your nurse also will give you an injection that will help you relax.

WHAT HAPPENS: Inside the x-ray room, you will lie flat on a table and a large, movable x-ray machine will be put into position just above you. The radiologist will decide which artery to use for the dye injection. Most often, the artery in the groin is chosen, but sometimes an artery in an arm may be used. Your skin will be shaved and cleaned and the doctor will inject a local anesthetic to numb the area; then he or she will wash the area with an antiseptic and surround it with sterile towels. The radiologist will put a needle into the artery and feed the catheter (along, thin, flexible tube) through the needle and through the entire length of the artery until it reaches the area to be examined. (Continuous x-ray pictures show the catheter's progress.) Then the doctor will inject the dye that will highlight the area in question and a series of x-ray pictures will be taken. When the catheter is removed, the doctor will apply firm pressure on your groin for at least 20 minutes to prevent bleeding. Then a thick, tight bandage will be placed over the area.

PAIN? DISCOMFORT: As the catheter moves through the blood vessel, you may feel it. It feels strange but very rarely painful. Many patients report considerable discomfort when the dye is injected into the blood stream. You may feel a hot, flushing sensation in your skin; you may notice a metallic taste in your mouth; you may feel sick to your stomach. These sensations rarely last more than 30 seconds. You also may start feeling restless and uncomfortable from lying on your back for a long time.

AFTERWARDS: You will have to stay flat in bed for 8 to 12 hours after the angiogram. You'll be asked to keep the bandaged leg or arm as straight as possible. For about 4 hours, a nurse will check your blood pressure, pulse, and temperature every 15 to 30 minutes. The nurse also will check your bandage for bleeding and will take your pulse in your foot or hand. As soon as you are stable, a nurse will take out the IV. After the first 4 hours, you will be checked less often, but you must still stay flat in bed. If the catheter entry point was in your arm, you will be allowed out of bed sooner. You can eat and drink again as soon as the test is finished. You should try to drink a full glass of water or juice every hour to help flush the dye out of your system. If the doctor decided to limit your fluids, the nurse will explain how much water you can drink. If you notice any bleeding or swelling at the catheter entry point, if you feel severe pain, or if your leg or arm starts to feel numb, be sure to report it to the nurse right away. With my permission the doctors proceeded to do the test. I was placed on the x-ray table in the supine position. I was having a fit with the pain in my foot and leg. The reason for this, was simple, I couldn't stand to elevate my leg up, because the circulation would completely stop in my foot and the lower part of my leg, and then the lower leg and the foot would begin to turn blue, and then the pain would get so bad, it would make the toughest man or woman alive shed tears. The doctors had to keep me drugged, in order to complete this test because I was going crazy due to the pain. The doctors had a hard time getting started with the test, but they finally got me in

Ferlin Clay Morgan

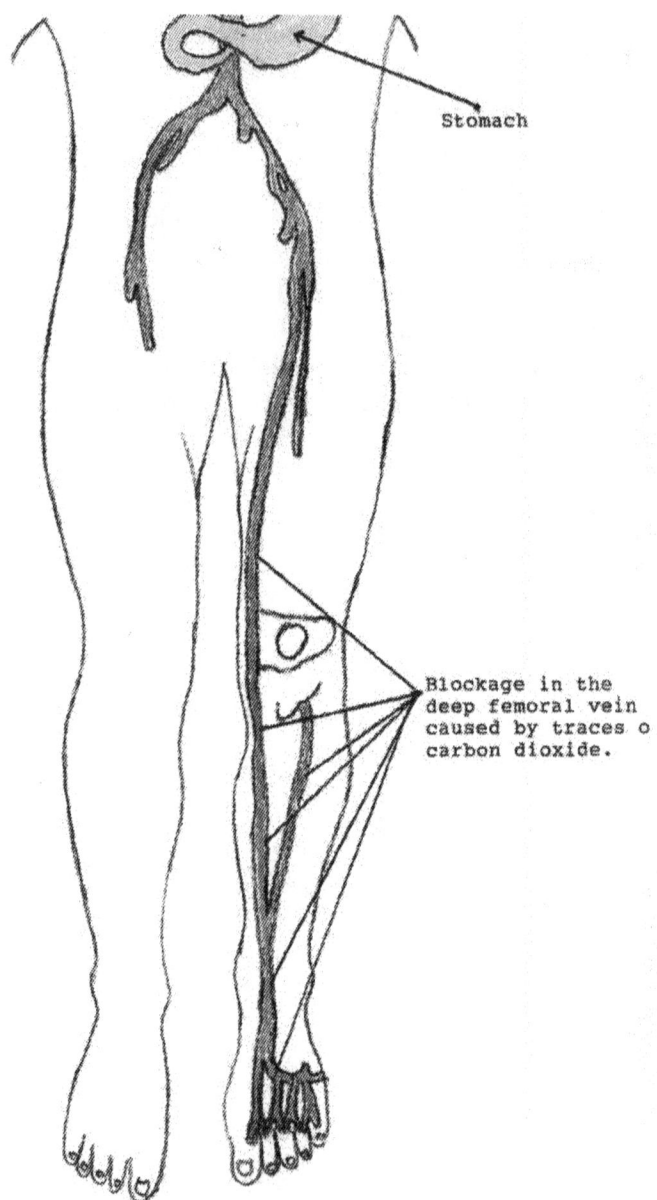

Stomach

Blockage in the
deep femoral vein
caused by traces o
carbon dioxide.

routine sterile fashion. The doctors said that Lidocaine 1% without Epinephringe was used for local anesthesia. Valium 10mg and Benadryl 50mg was given for IV sedation. (I was on a Demerol pump for pain control). Right femoral puncture was performed and catheter was advanced over guide wire into abdominal aorta. Following aortagram, catheter was advanced into the left iliac artery and a left lower extremity arteriogram was performed (including digital radiograph of the toes). The catheter was removed to the rightilioc artery for a right lower extremity exam. At this point of the testing the abdominal aorta and common ilioc arteries were normal. The doctors said on the left, the let common and external iliac artery were normal. The left superficial femoral artery as well as the popliteal arteries were normal. Below the knee, the peraneal artery was patent to just proximal to the ankle according to the doctors notes. Also the anterior and posterior tibial arteries terminate into thread like vessels in the mid calf. Digital examination of the left foot demonstrates thread like vessels in the left foot with no demonstrable digital artery. There was no evidence to suggest embolic disease. On the right, the right common and external iliac artery are widely patent. The right superficial femoral and popliteal artery were widely patent. Below the knee the peroneal artery was widely patent to the ankle with reconstitution of the posterior tibiol artery. The anterior tibiol artery terminates at the mid calf. The posterior tibiol artery terminates at the mid calf. When the doctors finished the Arteriorgram they said that there impression was as follows. 1. Markedly abnormal exam with occlusive disease involving each lower extremity, (left greater than the right) with both anterior and both posterior tibiol vessels terminating at mid calf. Each peroneal artery is patent (right greater than the left). 2. No evidence to suggest embolic disease. 3. Differential would include Thermal injury, Buergers disease, or other vasculitis, and less likely infections etiology. Clinical correction is suggested. After the arteriogram was finished I was taken back to my room, and that was where I had to lay flat on my back for about 4 to 6 hours, so that the puncture that was made in the right femoral artery, could have a chance to stop bleeding. After I was placed, into my room, I was told that it was lunch time. I was pretty hungry but I don't have a clue of what caused me to have such an appetite after the arteriogram test was finished. My wife told me that she had never seen me eat like that before. It was just as if I couldn't get enough of food to eat. But I couldn't remember how much I had ate. The wife said that I had ate one tray of food and then ask for another tray of food. According to my wife I also had ate part of her food that she had went out to the restaurant and picked up for herself. I do remember eating a lot of food, but there was something's that I couldn't remember, because I wasn't completely stable, due to the anesthesia that was given to me during the arteriogram testing. That pretty much summed up the day for me, other than getting an x-ray done later in the day. For the next few days I just laid around and took in some antibiotics to fight any infection that could be hanging around. The surgeon that admitted me into the hospital, on the first night that I showed up at the vascular surgeons office had to go out of town for about a week, so he turned me over to another surgeon, and a good surgeon at that. He come up to my room to talk to me about my surgery and to also tell the wife and I when and where and what time that he would like to perform the surgery. He scheduled my surgery for December 20, 1996 at 7:30 a.m. He also told me that he had discussed my situation with the other vascular doctors and reviewed the notes of the doctor that I had before him. He said that there was some consideration that I might have a Buerger's type of disease or severe distal peripheral vascular disease. Treatment options for me were discussed and based on non-invasive studies that I might be able to heal a transmetatorsal amputation and most certainly a below-knee amputation. However, because of my strong desire, the surgeon said that he would attempt to try a local procedure, by performing a distal amputation along to see if this would heal. The surgeon told me that there was also a strong possibility this may not heal, but I still wished to proceed with only a digital amputation. As bad as I wanted to hurry and get the surgery over with, I also dreaded it to. The night before my surgery I wasn't allowed to drink or eat after twelve o'clock. The nurses told the wife and I, pretty much everything that we needed to know about what we should do the morning before the surgery. I don't think the wife and I either one got any sleep the night before my surgery. I remember watching the clock that night, every chance that I could get. I wanted time to pass by real fast, but on the other hand I wanted time to pass by really slow. Regardless, it still seem like time passed by fast and it was 7:00 a.m. already and that wasn't good, because it was time for my surgery. I had to start getting myself ready. But with the wife's help it wasn't to bad. Around 6:30 a.m. a nurse came to my room and checked the IV in my arm and then she said that I needed a new one. When she said that I just set quietly and got very, very weak. The reason for this was simply because I had been poked so many times already with IV needles that I just couldn't take anymore. When the nurse attempted to change the IV, I was ready to fight, but I just didn't have the energy to do anything. They had to change the IV in my arm and I understood that, but my arms were sore and blue all over, and I just couldn't take any more pain. As the nurse was trying to get my IV changed these two old boys came through the door and saved the day. They were there to take me down for my surgery, and one of the boys told the nurse to just wait on the IV, because they can do it down in surgery, by numbing the area before the IV is put in the arm. The understanding that I got was, that the nurses out on the floor working wasn't permitted to do any kind of local blocking with such things as lidocaine. The only way that this hospital would let this happen would be if some one was sent up from surgery to your room and did this for the nurse. When I was taken down to surgery I must admit there was no pain at all when they changed my IV in my arm. When I reached the area where they changed my IV, this was like a holding room I believed. But anyway one of the staff members brought me a little bit of water and two pills to take. I did what I was told to do and that was to lay down and rest because it would be a little while before they would get to me. When I laid my head back on the pillow that was the last thing that I could remember. The two pills that I took just flat foot turned my light out, and in order to find out what happened during surgery I had to turn to my doctor's notes in order to find out every detail that happened other than what my doctor and my wife had told me. The doctor's notes would read as follows. The patient was taken to the operating room and placed on the operating table in the supine position. Because of the anxiety, the patient had pain in his left foot, general anesthesic was chosen. After induction of this, the left foot and toes were prepped with Betadine solution and dropped in a sterile fashion. An incision was placed around the base of the left second and third toes to include any necrotic tissue present. This was deepened through the subcutaneous tissue sharply and down to the level of the phalanx. The second and third digits were then removed at the junction of the metatarsal – phalangeal joint. The toes were then passed off as a specimen. There was fairly good bleeding from the skin edges and this was controlled by using electroautery. Wound was irrigated with antibiotic-containing solution. Because of prominence of the second metatorsal head, a limited debridgement with a rongeur was done. The bone appeared healthy and had good bleeding from its end. The subcutaneous tissue were approximated using three Vicryl sutures placed in interrupted fashion. The skin edge was then approximated using a combination of two and three nylon sutures placed in interrupted Vertical mattress fashion. There was some mild tension across the wound but the edges did approximate nicely without severe tension. Betedine ointment was applied to the wound and sterile dressing was applied. The foot was then wrapped with a Kerlix roll. The patient was extubated in the operating room and taken to the recovery room in stable condition. The patient tolerated the procedure well. There were no complications known during surgery. Estimated blood loss was 50cc Findings during surgery. There was fair blood supply to the skin and surrounding

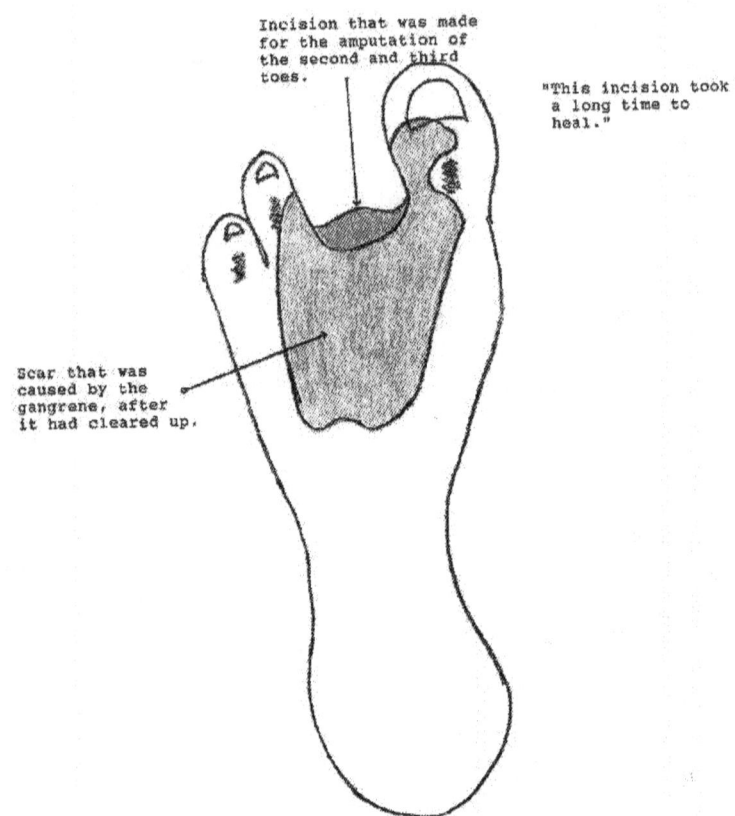

Incision that was made for the amputation of the second and third toes.

"This incision took a long time to heal."

Scar that was caused by the gangrene, after it had cleared up.

tissue of the left second and third toes. There was no necrotic tissue other than the gangrenous tissue in the toes themselves. The base of the toes appeared some what pale but did have fair perfusion. No other abnormalities were identified, during or after surgery. "That was pretty interesting now wasn't it." Sure it was! Well let's move along. I remember waking up in the recovery room, and I also remember what caused me to wake up, I was laying flat on my back, and as you remember, earlier in this book,

I talked about this! When I would lay down flat on my back or just lay down, my foot would feel like it was going to explode, and also there was the excruciating evil pain that hurt so badly that I would have assumed to die than to go through such an ordeal ever again in my life time. So you could imagine what I was thinking when I woke up. The pain was B.A.D., really bad before I had surgery, and for it to be hurting after surgery, I just knew that of all that I had went through, that the surgery hadn't done anything to help me and I just knew I would have to live or die with this evil pain. When I woke up I wasn't completely stable, even thou I thought I was. That is why I had these doubts of how or did the surgery even help me. I wasn't really thinking straight for a few moments, and then suddenly it hit me. I needed to hang my foot down over the side of the bed, and it would quit hurting. When I made an attempt to do this, the nurses ran over to stop me. Because of the risk of me falling out of my bed, and or tearing the sutures back loose in my foot. I remember talking out loud asking for my wife over and over, because I was having a fit with the pain in my foot. All of a sudden up walks one of the surgeons, and he ask me what was going on, and I told him that I wanted my wife, so she could help me drop my foot over the side of the bed, so that it would quit hurting. Guess what, the surgeon told me to go a head and drop my foot over the side of the bed very slow like. He held my foot until I got it where I wanted it, and then he ask me if the pain was easing up any, and I said yes. I think this stunned everybody that was in the recovery room. The reason why I think this, because when I was brought up from surgery I was still asleep, and for the first couple of hours everything was OK. And then as I started waking up

I began to cry out in pain with my foot. The understanding that I got was that I cried out in my sleep for over a half hour, before I woke up. There was some talk about keeping me in the intensive care until for the rest of the day, so that I could be closely watched after. But after everyone saw that I had settled down, including the surgeons, I was then moved back to my room out on the floor in the hospital. That's where I stayed from December 20, 1996 through December 24, 1996. After I was moved back out on the floor the only thing that I could do was wait a few days and hope and pray to God that when the surgeon comes to my room to examine my foot, that he tells me that it is showing progress of healing, and it's doing great. Because that would increase my chances of getting out of the hospital, and the wife and I would be able to go home and spend Christmas with our beautiful little boy. Well a few days had past by and the surgeon had examined my foot for the first time since my surgery, and he said that he couldn't see very much improvement at this time. This first follow up examination was on December 22, 1996 and my surgery took place on December 20, 1996. The surgeon said that he would like to keep me in the hospital for a couple more days, to see if the foot would show more signs of healing. Well for those two days, I just laid around and eat a lot and watched TV. I didn't have a lot of visitors during my stay in the hospital. But I did have my wife there with me, and it doesn't get any better than that. The wife and I wished that we could have had our little boy with us, but it just wasn't the time or place for him to be so he stayed with the wife's parents for the nine days that I was in the hospital. The wife had contacted several family members for me to see if they would come by and see me before my surgery, because if some thing happen to me during surgery, like maybe losing my leg or both legs, or possibly death. I wanted my family to hear the results of my surgery from the surgeon for themselves, rather than my wife being put in the position to deal with all the pressure, from my family if something bad was to happen to me during surgery. It was December 24, 1996 in the late afternoon hours, when the surgeon returned to my room again, to examine my foot for the second time since my surgery on December 20, 1996. When the surgeon finished the examination of my foot this time around, he said that he believed that I could heal a local amputation after further examination of my foot. He said that he was concerned about this, earlier due to the poor noninvassion and arteriogream findings in both lower extremities. I strongly preferred to attempt a digital amputation alone, and if this should fail, then a transmetatarsol. There was talk about a below-the-knee amputation if the transmetatorsal failed to heal. I just had a good feeling about the digital amputation. I had to doctor my foot every day and observe its changes for better than a year and a half, before I found a doctor that made a lot of since to me when he would tell me what he believed was going on with my foot. The two toes, alone turned black, but the gangrene, that was on my foot did heal up. Thanks to the foot doctor that I had seen for a couple months. He was the one, if you remember that gave me the 7 day dosage of prednisone to help heal up the gangrene on my foot. After doing so, if you recall he referred me over to the Vascular surgeons for a possible amputation of the second and third toes. During the time I was taking the prednisone, to heal up the gangrene, the two blackened toes tried to heal up quite a bit themselves also.

So as you can see, I had a strong feeling that a digital amputations alone would heal up. But there was still some thoughts in my head, of whether or not that the cramps and pains in my legs would get better to with the digital amputation, and the clearing of the infection in my body. Well my question was answered a few months later, after my surgery. The pains that I was having in my legs was for sure gone, but the cramps were still there with occasional pain in the left foot. I also still had the bad pains in both arms, plus the back cramps that had bothered me for quite some time. It was believed to be the lack of blood flow that I had in my legs and feet, due to the damaged arteries, and small vessels in the lower part of my legs and feet. Well regardless of my opinion the surgeon had his opinion about my surgery to. He said that my postoperative course has been remarkable other than the significant pain initially after surgery I was taking in IV narcotics with a PCA pump for the first few days after my surgery. I subsequently had been able to be switched to oral narcotics and was doing fairly well, according to the surgeon. I told the surgeon as of the present time, that my foot feels better than it has in over a year. The surgeon told me that the wound is healing adequately. He also said there was some serious drainage from the wound, that is some times called joint water. Regardless of the drainage tissue present, and that was very good sign of healing. The surgeon said over all, the foot appears to be improving. I had been converted from IV antibiotics to PO antibiotics and was ambulating with crutches and still had significant pain in the foot when it was dependent.

Over all, I stated to the surgeon that the foot feels much better at this time, the surgeon felt that I was stable enough to be discharged to go home. I will say this much for the wife and I there couldn't have been any happier couple, when the surgeon said that he was going to let me go home. The surgeon said that he would like to see me back in his office in about two weeks from my discharge of the hospital. The surgeon said that if the foot is healing well when I return to his office that he would remove the sutures from my foot. The surgeon also told me to return to his office if I should notice increased redness, increased pain, fever, chills, or other signs of infection. The medications that I was discharged to go home with was Lortab plus one to two every 4 to 6 hours for pain, (#50).

Augmentin 500mg. One tablet three times a day for ten days. Prednisone 10mg. One tablet two times daily, for five days. At last the wife and I were homeward bound, and were so excited, because we were going to get to see our little boy finally, and we also would be in the comfort of our own home. But little that we knew, when we reached our home. We had decided to stop there first before we picked up our little boy from his grandparents house. As we began to enter our home, my wife open the door for me so that I could get through the door without hitting my foot over the door, but unlucky me cleared the door just fine, but after I got into our home, I bumped my foot over the entertainment center. I didn't have a leg rest on my wheel chair, so I had to ambulate on crutches and keep my leg and foot up level. This was very hard to do because the muscles in my left leg was very small and very weak, there for it was hard for me to hold my leg up level in front of me, and there absolutely was no way that I could drop my foot downward at that time, because of the pressure that would rush into my foot. It felt like my foot was swelling very rapidly and the pain would for sure make a grown man cry, regardless of how tough that he may be. Well anyway the wife and I entered our home, and we began to encounter a strong odor that smelt like soured mop water or something. The wife was more concerned of the hard lick that my foot took when I bumped it into the entertainment center, so she waited until she saw that I was alright, then she began to look for that bad odor, she didn't have to go very far to find out what the odor was. When she found it I wasn't to far away from her when she turned and told me that the water lines had froze and busted. And that we didn't have any water. It was then that I began to panic a little because I had to have the water to wash and soak my foot, so that it wouldn't get infected. My wife told me to not worry because she would get me some water one way or another. Bless her heart, she did just that. She carried water in from the neighbors house for about five days, before we could get the water lines repaired. Every water line in the house had froze and busted. And if that wasn't enough, after we had the water lines replaced, the repair man turned the water on and it was then, that we found out that the hot water tank had froze and busted to. The wife and I had the same thoughts in our head, and that what could possible happen to us next. We had very hard life for more than two years and we just couldn't understand why we were having all of this bad luck. We didn't have a very big Christmas at all, due to the water not working in the house, the wife couldn't prepare Christmas dinner for us, and even if she could have, she wouldn't have been able to clean up everything. Due to the substantial amount of time that I had to stay in the hospital and then being released on Christmas Eve, we were unable to do any Christmas shopping. But luckily my wife had picked up a few things for our little boy before I had been scheduled to go into the hospital for surgery. The wife and I noticed that our little boy had been under a lot of stress during the two weeks that we were gone to the hospital. When the wife went to pick our little boy up at his grandparents house, the wife said that he acted very odd, as if he was scared of her or was mad at us because we were gone for so long. It was a heart breaking experience for my wife, because she couldn't understand why our little boy was acting the way that he was. The wife would call him up by telephone and let him know, that we still loved him and that we would be home as soon as possible. That just proves that children sometimes may not show their feelings the way that we would expect them too, but most of all, it let the wife and I know just how much that our little boy had missed us. And it also reminded us just how much that our little boy depends on us to be there for him as his parents. During my first follow-up on my foot surgery, I was able to get a copy of my medical reports from the vascular surgeons office on my request. I had heard about everything that had took place during my surgery, and the results afterwards. But I had not heard any comments concerning a Surgical Pathology Report. When I received my medical records, the Pathologist Reports were in the stack of records to. The Pathology Report wasn't as bad as I figured it to be, as far as the reading goes. Even thou the report was very short in words, it just simply got straight to the point, of what anybody would want to know about the Pathology Report. Here is a little of what the Pathologist had to say about me in their report. The specimen was labeled second, third toes, left foot. Received in fixative were two toes connected by a small amount of skin and soft tissue of the foot. The toes measured 3.5x1.7x1.7cm and 4.2x1.8x1.7cm. They were partially covered by skin; however, the majority of the skin surface is soft, brown, beige and black in color, very flaky and foul smelling. Sectioning revealed underlying necrotic tissue. The majority of the cut surface of the distal ends of each toe was reddish-black. There were no toenails attached. Pathologist Diagnosis revealed as follows. Left 2nd and 3rd toes appear to be, focal fibrotic arterial occlusion. Ischemic necrosis and foci of acute inflammation. The Pathologist said that, despite of my age of 30 years, there were clear cut changes of Vascular occlusion and ischemic necrosis as well as the foci of marked acute inflammation in the soft tissue. The Vascular occlusions appeared to be by fibrous tissue which may have been an organized clot rather than ateroscerotic fibrous proliferation. My first scheduled follow up on the amputations of the left second and third toes, took place on January 1, 1997. The vascular surgeon began to examine my foot, and this is what the vascular surgeon had to say in his own words. This patient returns today for a scheduled follow up after undergoing amputations of the left second and third toes performed on December 20, 1996. The patient is only thirty years old and he has over a year long history of gangrenous changes to these toes, finally requiring amputation. His arteriogram shows extensive distal arterial disease suggestive of Buerger's Disease in both lower extremities. Fortunately, he had not had the problems with the right foot or toes. Options were discussed prior to surgery including possible transmetatarsal even below knee amputation. However, based on his young age and his strong desire to keep his foot intact, we told him that we would try a digital amputation alone. Noninvasive studies done preoperatively suggested poor digital pressures and we were worrisome that his might not heal. However, this was done in hopes of salvaging his foot. Upon returning today, the patient states overall he feels better. The patient still has significant pain in the region and there is still extreme tenderness at the amputation sites. The patient is able to walk on his right foot now, which he has not done for quite a while. The patient still has some soreness and weakness in the leg caused by the vascular disease. Over all, however, he was quite pleased. Patient denies any fever, chills, worsening of his amputation site or other problems. Patient reveals that the foot appears perfused. The patient has had breakdown and slumping of the skin over the amputation site leaving an area approximately 2 ½ to 3 centimeters long and 2 ½ to 3 centimeters wide in the gap between his first and fourth toes of the foot. There is some yellow fibrinous debris present, but underlying there appears to be healthy granulation tissue. This area appears to be getting smaller according to the patients account. It appears that although he did slough the superficial skin, he may be able to heal this area. The granulation tissue is healthy appearing and with minimal debridgement there appears to be adequate blood supply to the region. His sutures were still in place, although they were no longer holding skin together as this is sloughed. The sutures were removed with some difficulty because of local tenderness. There is no erythema or evidence of significant purulent drainage from the area.

Ferlin Clay Morgan

IMPRESSION: 1.   Status post amputations of left second and third toes with subsequent skin sloughing – stable.
2.   Bilateral lower extremity distal arterial disease – possible Buerger's Disease.
3.   Is previous tobacco user, but patient has quit.

PLAN: 1.   I have encouraged the patient to continue local care to the area. There is good granulation tissue present. I am hopeful that the area will contract down and finally heal. I have asked him to begin soaking the foot twice a day as tolerated. The foot still has significant tenderness but if he can tolerate rinsing this two to three times a day, it may help this area to heal faster. I have also written him a prescription for Silvadene cream which may provide some soothing benefit to the area. I have also written a prescription for Percocet 1 to be taken every 4 to 6 hours as needed for pain. The Lortab Plus he had been taking is not controlling his pain as well as he would like. I will plan to see the patient back in two weeks or sooner if he should have problems.

Patient has returned 01/21/97 for scheduled follow up after undergoing amputations of the left second and third toes performed on 12/20/96. The patient had significant distal arterial disease suggestive of Buerger's disease. He was last seen here on 01/07/97 at which time there had been some sloughing of the skin but overall adequate of the amputation sites. Upon return today the states he feels well. He still has significant pain in the region but it appears to be improving. He states he is able to rest at night which he was unable to do for twelve to eighteen months prior to his surgery. He states he still has some pain in the foot in the mornings and it is difficult for him to walk on the left foot but overall he does feel better. He denies any fever, chills or worsening of the ulceration on his foot. Physical examination reveals perhaps some gradual improvement with closing down in the skin edges at the left second and third toe amputation sites. There is still a relatively deep ulceration present with some fibrinopurulent debris present in the base. A couple of Vicryl sutures are visible in the wound. The remainder of the foot is pink and appears adequately perfused. There does not appear to be worsening of the area of ulceration. I did some superficial debridgement in the office with removal of the two remaining Vicryl sutures. Also some of the excess fibrinopurulent debris was lightly debrided. Patient cannot tolerate extensive debridgement because of sensitivity and pain in the region.

IMPRESSION:
1. Status post amputation of left second and third toes for gangrenous changes –stable.
2. Bilateral lower extremity distal arterial disease – possible Buerger's disease; patient is a previous tobacco user- denies use at present time.

PLAN:
1. I have asked the patient to continue his local wound care with the twice daily washings of his left foot and application of Silvadene cream. I will plan to see him back in two weeks for follow up. I will be happy to see him prior to that if he should have increasing pain or worsening of his wound. He may still require further debridgement and/or amputation at the transmetatarsal or even the below knee level if this does not heal.

Patient returns today February 4, 1997 for a follow up after undergoing amputations of the left second and third toes performed on December 20, 1996. He was last seen here on January 21, 1997, at which time, the amputation sites were making slow, but adequate progress. Please recall, the patient had evidence of significant arterial disease in both lower extremities, being worse on the left. This is certainly suggestive of Berger's Disease.

Overall, today, he feels well. He still has pain at the amputation site, but this appears to be primarily at night and it is a tingling pain. We have discussed the use of Elavil in the past, but apparently he had a bad experience with Elavil and does not desire to retake it. The pain in his left foot is decreasing and overall he feels well. He thinks that the opened area of granulation tissue is slowing closing in.

PHYSICAL EXAMINGATION: I agreed with the patient that there is a decrease in the size of the opened area where the left second and third toes used to be. There is excellent pranulation tissue present. Some yellow fibrinous debris was easily removed in the office today and underneath this is healthy granulation tissue. The skin edges are contracted down overall the opened wound is significantly smaller in size. The remainder of the left foot appears well perfused with good capillary refill. I can not palpate pedal pulses, but this is not unchanged from previous exams.

IMPRESSION:
1. Amputations of the left second and third toes for gangrenous changes – slowly improving.
2. Bilateral lower extremity arterial disease – possible Berger's disease. Patient is a previous tobacco user but hasn't used tobacco since hospitalization in December.

PLAN:
1. I have asked the patient to continue his local wound care with twice daily washings of his left foot and application of Silvadene cream. He is doing an excellent job at home and I have asked him to continue this. I will plan to see him back in one month for follow up appointment. He may return sooner if he

has worsening of his pain or any problems with his wound. He is pleased with his progress so far and because he is symptomatically improving, I feel it is reasonable to continue. If he should have worsening of his symptoms or pain consideration should be given to trasmetataral or even blow knee amputation.

This patient returns today March 4, 1997 for re-evaluation of the amputated on December 20, 1996 for gangrenous changes to these toes. Prior to surgery he underwent work up which was highly suggestive of Buerger's disease. The toes were amputated and there was concern at the time that this area would not heal and that he would not even heal a transmetatarsal amputation site. However because of his age we thought it was a worthwhile attempt.

Since that time the area has been healing adequately. In fact, I have been somewhat surprised that the area has healed as quickly as it has. The patient states today that the area is much less tender that it has been and he is quite pleased with the improvement since he was here one month ago. Examination reveals continued closure of the area at the base of the left second and third toes (amputation site). The area is much less tender and overall is contracting down nicely. There is fibrinopurulent debris at the base of this area but there is underlying healthy pink granulation tissue. The tenderness is markedly decreased from what it was one month ago. The remainder of the foot appears well perfused with good capillary refill.

IMPRESSION:
1. Open area at the base of the left second and third toe amputation sites – slowly improving.
2. Status post left second and third toe amputations performed on December 20, 1996.
3. Bilateral lower extremity arterial disease – probably Buerger's disease. Patient has a history of being a previous tobacco abuser but none at present time.

PLAN:
1. The patient is doing well. I have asked him to continue with the local wound care that he has been providing. I expect this area will continue to close down. I will plan to see him back in one month.
2. I have written the patients prescriptions for Penicillin Vee-K 500 milligrams to be taken four times a day. Tylenol #3 one to be taken every three to four hours as needed for pain.

This patient returns today April 8, 1997 for scheduled follow up an pre-evaluation of the left second and third toe amputation sites. Please recall, patient underwent amputations of the left second and third toes on December 20, 1996 for progressive gangrenous changes. Preoperative evaluation strongly suggested Buerger's disease. I was doubtful that this area would heal but fortunately this area has slowly been healing in.

Upon return today he states he feels well. He is walking much better as the pain is leaving the foot. He is pleased with the healing of his amputation site.

PHYSICAL EXAMINATION: Continued closure of the amputation site at the left second and third toes. There is healthy granulation tissue present and the wound is much smaller than it was when I last saw him on March 4, 1997. There is good granulation tissue present in the base and the area is closing quite nicely. I thought I may have felt a faint dorsalis pedis pulse but I would be surprised if this was the case simply because of his severe distal disease noted on previous vascular studies and arteriogram.

IMPRESSION:
1. Continued healing of an open area at the base of the left second and third toe amputation sites.
2. Left second and third toe amputations performed on December 20, 1996.
3. Bilateral lower extremity arterial disease – probable Buerger's disease, patient is a previous tobacco user-no tobacco use at present time. (None since surgery).

The patient continues to do well. I will plan to see him back in the office in six weeks. He may return sooner if he should have any problems. I expect he will continue to do well.

SUBJECTIVE: Patient has returned today May 20, 1997 for scheduled follow up after undergoing amputations of his left second and third toes, which was performed on December 20, 1996. This was done for probable Berger's disease. He was last seen here on April 4, 1997, at which time the area was healing nicely. It was somewhat of a surprise that he would heal this area at all based on his preoperative non-invasive studies and arteriograms, however, he has done nicely. Upon return today, he states he is doing well. The area continues to close down. The discomfort he was having at the site continues to improve. The open area of the wound continues to heal down and is almost completely closed. He has a faintly palpable dorsalis pedis pulse and his toes are well-perfused and they actually have hair on the remaining toes of the left foot.

IMPRESSION:
1. Continued healing of open area at the base of left second and third toe amputation sites.
2. Status post left second and third toe amputations performed on December 20, 1996.
3. Bilateral lower extremity arterial – probable Buerger's disease. Patient still hasn't used tobacco since surgery.

PLAN:
1. The patient will continue his local wound care. I plan to see him back in 6 weeks. He may return sooner if he should have any problems.

Patient has returned today July 1, 1997 for scheduled follow-up after undergoing amputations of his left second and third toes, which was performed on December 20, 1996. The patient is wearing a loose fit shoe, something he says that he hasn't done in over 18 months, not to mention the fact that the patient is walking on the left foot now. Something that the patient says that he also hasn't done in over a year, without the help of crutches. The wound has closed down completely, and has done very nicely as far as the healing process goes. He states that there is pain in the area of the wound that is really bad at times. I told the patient that this would go away with time, because it usually takes about two year's for a wound like this to get back to about 80%, and for it to quit bothering him with pain. I plan to see the patient in 6 weeks, if he feels that I need to see him again. The patient may return sooner if he should have any problems.

The six week's had past and I was doing very well as far as the healing process goes, but there was some pain and swelling that remained in the foot and leg. As of this day the foot still isn't completely 100% pain free. Actually the foot still hurts a lot, and swells when I lay down at night to sleep. I also have a lot of pain with my foot, when bad weather sets in for a little while. About two months after the surgery was performed to amputate the two toes, I began to wear a shoe on my foot, something that I hadn't done in a long time. I had wondered for about a year and a half if, I would ever be able to set my weight back on my left foot ever again. I guess that if I hadn't been so determined to walk on my foot, I may have never walked on my left foot as of this day, because I had to deal with a lot of severe pain in my foot and leg both at the same time. The area where the amputation was performed was very painful, due to the debridgement or smoothing of the bone where the left second and third toes were amputated. I also

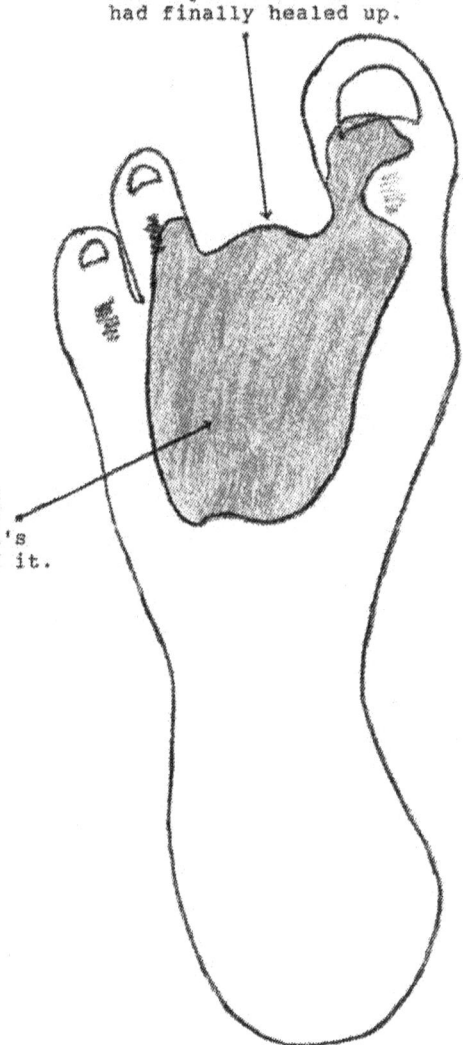

The outer surface of the amputation incision had finally healed up.

The gangrene had defiantly healed up. With no sign's of recurrence of it.

had a lot of pain in the muscles of the left foot and leg, because I hadn't used the muscles in that foot and leg in over a year and a half. The muscles in the left leg and foot felt like they had been pulled or sprained really bad, and the pains that I was having didn't seem like they were ever going to stop. I also was dealing with a lot of other troubling pains to, at that time. As you recall, I had been taking narcotic medication for a long time, actually long enough that it's probably safe to say that, I was addicted to the narcotic pills. But, I also was determined to get off of the narcotics, so I proceeded to do so. For about four to five days in a row, it simply felt like my body was going to come apart. It literally felt like the muscles in my body were being stretched and torn apart. I overcome the addition of the narcotic pills and the pain that you have, when you quit taking the narcotic pills. The next painful addiction problem, I had to face following the narcotics addiction, was the addition of cigarettes. All smokers will tell basically the same story, as far as quitting cigarettes goes. If you go to long without a cigarette, you'll get really nervous and very edgy, and if you don't get a cigarette soon, you feel like your going to loose control of yourself. About two days after, I had quit smoking, I began to have wearied feelings all over, that felt like little beebee's running all through my body. This also seemed to occur when I would take a deep breath of air into my lungs. Even after the wearied feelings had past it still took about two and a half to three weeks to get past the cramps and pains after I had quit smoking cigarettes. But now as far as having the really bad cravings for a cigarette goes, it took me around six months, I guess to be able to really say that I had control of those bad cravings. To be sure that no one gets a misunderstanding of what I mean by saying I have control over those bad cravings for cigarettes, is that I can now say that it has been two years now since I gave up smoking cigarettes, and I don't feel like I'm going to go out of my mind for the need of a cigarette. The vascular surgeon diagnosed me, to be suffering from bergers disease. This disease has been found to be a direct link to cigarette smoking. This disease was the blame for all my troubles that I was suffering with in the past. Such as the inflamed veins and blood clots that I had in my legs. These same blood clots closed of the circulation in my foot, and that's when my foot began to swell with a lot of inflammation. Little that I knew at the time, but the inflammation had spreaded through out my hole body, and it was then, that I encountered a lot of different body pains. Such as the muscle fatigue, head aches, back pain. Chest pains, pain in my hips, pain in my arms, all of the severe sinus infections. Loss of appetite, ear infections, tooth ache. Just name one, I've had to deal with several body pains in the past. But I think without a doubt in mind, that the pain that I had with my foot, when the gangrene had set up in it, was the worst pain of all. But when all was said and done for, I think I was very lucky to lose only the two toes and to end up with the Fibromyalgia arthritis In my nervous system. I could have been on the unlucky end of the deal, and lost a lot more than just the two toes. I could have just as easily lost my foot, or more so, I could have lost my complete leg during all of this. A little better than two years has past since, I had to have surgery on my foot, and I still haven't used any kind of tobacco products. In fact I'm glad that I was able to quit smoking, because I didn't really realize how much of my life was taken away from me, when I was a smoker. I've noticed that I can hear better, everything that I eat has a better taste. I have also noticed that a lot of things smell better to. Such things as flowers, foods, and drinks, just about anything that could be thought of. I'm truly glad that God gave me the strength to quit smoking. Because it has definitely been a plus for me. I trust that anyone, person that reads this story, and that if she or he is a smoker, that they will strongly consider to quit smoking. Before I finish the last page of this excruciating story, I would like to express my appreciation to everyone that believed in me, and stood strongly beside me and that helped me get through those two very long but stressful, and painful, life threatening years. Beginning with my wife, thank you for being there for me, in my time of need, and that I can for ever say that you took your wedding vows serious, because you stuck with me through sickness and in health and for better or for worse, and I love you for that. I also would like to say thank you to my wife, for finding the time to be the perfect mother, for our little boy during these bad times. I don't have a clue to how you was able to keep yourself going during those two very long excruciating years, but I am sure glad that you stuck it out with me, because I don't know how our little boy and I could have made it without you. Just remember in our eyes, and thoughts you was, the perfect mother and wife back then, and you are still the perfect mother and wife as of this day. Our little boy and I think you are the greatest and we love you, don't ever forget that. I would like to take time to say, that I appreciate all the doctors and their staff members, that made an effort to cure my illnesses and never prevailed. I also would like to say thank you to the foot doctor that helped me, when I needed help in the worst of times, I can't thank you enough it was you that saved my foot, when you cleared up the wet gangrene, that covered the top of my foot. Once again, I would like to say thank you, and that nor yourself or your work will ever be forgotten. Last but not the least of all, to the Vascular Surgeons that I have nicknamed the magnificent 5. You all are without a doubt the best that the wife and I have ever seen in your profession. You all could have easily took me into surgery and done a simple amputation of the two toes, but you all went further than that. I was placed on antibiotics for about 5 days to get some of the swelling down due to the inflammation and the infection in my foot. The 5 days of antibiotics ease the pain in my foot, and that was a big relief for me. There several test that was performed on me for a lot of different things. Such as the pressure test and a Doppler test was done on my legs. Then you all had x-rays taken of my lungs, and an arteriolgram performed to locate the blockages in my legs. All of this was performed very professionally like, and then I was taken to surgery. Everyone handled their jobs like professionals and everything moved along just like clock work during surgery, and now I am doing really well. Well enough, that I am walking every day on my foot now, and I am very, very happy. I would like to express my appreciation to those 5 Vascular surgeons by saying I thank you, and that I will never forget you all and for what you all have done for me. "Thank you".